Helen Giles

From Kitchen
to Consumer

From Kitchen to Consumer

THE ENTREPRENEUR'S GUIDE TO COMMERCIAL FOOD PRODUCTION

Barbara Nelson Stafford

Wyoming Department of Commerce
Division of Economic and Community Development
Cheyenne, Wyoming

With Susan Koster

ACADEMIC PRESS, INC.
Harcourt Brace Jovanovich, Publishers
San Diego   New York   Boston   London
Sydney   Tokyo   Toronto

This book is intended as a resource for entrepreneurs interested in exploring
the food processing industry. It provides generally applicable information on
a variety of topics, including legal matters, regulatory compliance, accounting, and tax. It is not intended to provide professional advice in these or other
areas, and the entrepreneur is responsible for obtaining appropriate advice
and information with regard to these matters. Each business is different, and
the entrepreneur must use his or her own judgment about any matter
pertaining to the operation of the business. Therefore, neither the author nor
the publisher can assume any liability for any actions undertaken as a result
of the information presented in this book.

Academic Press, Inc.
San Diego, California 92101

United Kingdom Edition published by
Academic Press Limited
24–28 Oval Road, London NW1 7DX

Library of Congress Cataloging-in-Publication Data

Nelson-Stafford, Barbara, date
    From kitchen to consumer : the entrepreneur's guide to commercial
food production / Barbara Nelson-Stafford.
        p.   cm.
    ISBN 0-12-662770-3
    1. Food industry and trade--Management.   2. New business
enterprises--Management.   3. Entrepreneurship.   I. Title.
HD9000.5.S67   1991
664'0068--dc20   91-11604
                                                        CIP

PRINTED IN THE UNITED STATES OF AMERICA
91 92 93 94   9 8 7 6 5 4 3 2 1

This book is dedicated to my children, Melissa and Ben Nelson, for their patience and understanding during all the years of living with a working mom, and to my husband, Bill Stafford, for providing a nurturing environment from which this book grew.

Special thanks to Jim and Elliot and all my friends for putting up with me during my "writing time."

Contents

APPENDIX A

APPENDIX B

APPENDIX C

APPENDIX D

APPENDIX E

Preface

In the food industry it is known as "The Great Gamble." In any given year, over 10,000 new products make it to the grocer's shelves. Unfortunately, only a small percentage of these new products make it through the first year and less than 1% will be available within 3 years of the initial placement. As any industry executive will tell you, it's a tough business.

A large number of these new products are developed through the efforts of the Research and Development (R&D) departments of the food "giants." These major conglomerates, such as General Foods, Nestlé, and Ralston Purina, to name a few, are rapidly increasing in size as the food industry satiates its endless appetite for merger and acquisition. These major food companies can afford aggressive R&D facilities staffed by innovative food-processing experts who constantly develop prototypes of new products. They also have the "deep pockets" required to launch major national marketing and advertising programs to support these new products, and the potential profitability of one or two successful new product lines justifies the cost. With the proper amount of capital and professional support, somehow it seems to all work out.

This book has been developed to assist the other major competitive player in the food industry—the undercapitalized, less-than-technically astute, usually understaffed, business person who is also trying to launch that elusive entity, the "successful" food product line. If you are an entrepreneur who has a product and a strong desire to see it produced in mass market quantities, safely entrenched and desired on the shelves of supermarkets all over the country, you are not alone! Each year thousands of people all over the world take the plunge and develop a food business. Unfortunately, most of them are attempting this task through sheer trial and error, unaware of the plethora of excellent federal, state, and locally sponsored programs available to assist them in their endeavor. Too often the assistance they need is requested *after* they have spent every bit of available working capital and when they are one step away from bankruptcy.

It is my sincere hope that you will take the time to read through this book *before* you start spending your, and possibly your friends', hard earned money. Wise decisions from the onset will give you a competitive edge in this tough business.

This book offers a simple, step-by-step guide to developing a value-added food product business. It is a tool to *assist* you in your efforts and should be treated as such. Throughout the text you will be advised when you need to seek assistance and where it is available. There are excellent programs throughout the country sponsored by such groups as the Small Business Administration (SBA), federal and state Departments of Agriculture, universities, and local community colleges, just to name a few, who are waiting to assist you. Most of these programs offer professional counseling support in all aspects of developing your food processing business—usually at no cost to the business person. They are listed by state or region throughout the book—use them! There will come a time, particularly during your start-up phase, when the services of a qualified professional (such as a tax accountant or business lawyer) will be required. Spending money wisely for the right type of assistance will save you hassles and dollars in the long run. In this book I have tried to assist you in identifying the type of professional you need, the type of questions to ask, and how to locate the best person in your geographic location.

The information is here. If you take time to read and follow the guidelines, you are sure to increase your chances of reaching your goal of becoming a successful, value-added food producer.

The majority of credit for the information regarding resources and strategies for the entrepreneur contained in this book goes to the United States Small Business Administration (SBA). The SBA has long been the primary federal resource for the small business person and their efforts are to be commended. The quality and quantity of pertinent information available through SBA offices around the country is invaluable to anyone seriously considering starting a business.

I would also like to acknowledge the University of Colorado Business Advancement Centers (CUBAC) for the use of several of their excellent small business worksheets. The staff of CUBAC has been instrumental in developing simplified data and worksheets to assist the entrepreneur in his or her business development stages. Patty Martillero, Karen Eye, and the staff of CUBAC have been a constant source of support, not only for myself, but for business people throughout the state of Colorado.

The following organizations should be recognized for the excellent resources they make available to the small business person, as noted throughout this book: the United States Department of Commerce; United States Department of Agriculture; Federal Drug Administration; Internal Revenue Service; Uniform Product Code Council; AT&T; Bank of America; and Coopers and Lybrand, Inc.

Finally, I would like to acknowledge the Wyoming Division of Economic and Community Development for their support during the completion of this book.

Introduction

Since the beginning of civilization, humans have had a desire to process food. Two hundred and fifty thousand years ago, Peking Man used fire to cook his food. This could be considered one of the earliest forms of food processing. Through some accident, no doubt, raw animal flesh was dropped on or near a fire. When primitive man discovered that roasted meat had a different texture and flavor and, more importantly, spoiled less readily, the food processing industry was launched!

Food processing was a very strong industry during Roman times. In fact, one of the major reasons for the aggressive expansion of the Roman Empire was to obtain more food for Italy. In particular, the grapes from France, Austria, Germany, Hungary, and Rumania were absolutely necessary for Italian wine production.

The bureaucrats got into the act (and stayed in, as you will see when we discuss local, state, and federal regulations regarding food processing) between the thirteenth and sixteenth centuries. During that period, all the major branches of the food industry in the civilized world became subject to detailed regulations designed to protect the consumer.

During the Middle Ages, commercial food processing and preservation became more developed, leading to less and less home food preparation.

Obviously, the impact of the Industrial Revolution on food production was enormous. More sophisticated methods of food processing were developed, as well as a much more efficient system of transportation.

Another milestone for food processing was the commercial development, by a gentleman named Appert, of the canning process in the eighteenth century.

Today, the latest developments in science and engineering usually have some application in food processing.

You are about to become involved in one of the most exciting, rapidly changing industries in the world—that of food processing!

CHAPTER 1

Choosing the Right Product

So you want to be a food processor? Why? Is the world breaking down your door, trying to get a mason jar of your "secret" barbecue sauce? Did your Aunt Sarah leave you the only copy of her extra-special jelly recipe? Are your famous chocolate chip cookies always the first to be sold out at the church bake sale? It seems that everybody knows someone who makes *the best* sauce or *the best* chili seasoning. It's nice to know that something that you prepare especially for your family and friends is so well received but, believe me, the idea of mass marketing a favorite recipe is usually not a reason to mortgage the farm. There are, of course, exceptions to the rule: Take, for instance, Mrs. Fields, Famous Amos, or Mo Siegel of Celestial Seasonings Herb Tea fame. Let's not forget Paul Newman and his popcorn, salad dressing, and spaghetti sauce products. Keep in mind that Paul had a bit of a promotional advantage when his picture appeared on each bottle.

A bit of skepticism or caution at this stage of your planning process can save you a lot of aggravation and money in the long run. When you are trying to decide what kind of product or product line you would like to being producing, it's important that you remember that competing against the food giants (Kraft, General Foods, Swanson, General Mills, Hunt-Wesson, etc.) is going to be very difficult unless you can compete on price or marketing dollars. If you do not have an effective way to cut

1

costs while maintaining quality, you are going to have a hard time convincing the average customer that your sauce is significantly better than the competition's product. If it is significantly better, you are going to need a great many marketing dollars to convince consumers that they should pay the extra money.

Okay, so you've decided that you *really* want to be a food processor. There are several ways to identify what type of product will be well received by the market and which will work for you.

Take a hard look at the types of products that are currently selling well in your regional grocery market. Try to strategize how you can expand on an existing concept to supply a new product with old consumer loyalties. For instance, make a product that is easier to use. Examples are microwave popcorn, instant muffin mix, and frozen pie crust. Try to develop a product that combines benefits, such as salad dressing containing vinegar and low-cholesterol oil, gravy mix with seasoning and thickening agents, or complete soup mixes. With the increased number of working mothers, women are constantly looking for convenience in their meal preparation. Although microwave cooking is leading the convenience trend, many women are looking for products which can be added to fresh meat and vegetables to save preparation steps and time.

Add something to a popular product. When a major beverage manufacturer decided to add 10 percent real fruit juice to one of its pop drink standards, it suddenly found that it was the largest selling fruit-flavored soft drink on the market. Adding NutraSweet® to several of its instant European coffee drinks created a whole new market niche for General Foods.

Figure out other uses for existing products. Consumers don't always use a product the way it was originally designed to be used. Remember what happened when baking soda (a generic cooking staple for decades) was suddenly marketed as a refrigerator deodorizer? What about the party mix you've been munching on for years that is an interesting mix of Chex breakfast cereal and whatever else might happen to be in your pantry that contains large quantities of salt? The new prepackaged Chex party mix is being enthusiastically received by a consumer base that has known about it for years—now it's just more convenient.

Take something out of an existing product. For instance, look how popular the caffeine-free colas are becoming. There are new products popping up daily that have less salt, less sugar, less oil, and less calories. Consumers are looking for old favorites that are healthier for them.

Think of something that copies a substitute product. For example, pet owners constantly feed their animals table scraps to supplement the perceived blandness of common dried pet food products. Gourmet pet products which are competitively priced have great consumer appeal. Adding dried gravy flavoring, eggs, or cheese to dried dog food is usually not cost prohibitive and provides a new product niche.

Appeal to the child in every adult or to every mother's concern for her children's healthy food intake. Think of the hundreds of new ice cream novelties flooding the market. Dole fruit bars took the basic popsicle concept, added real fruit juices, reduced sugar, and became an instant success with young, healthy, nutrition-minded adults.

Go to food shows. Every food show, both in the United States and overseas, features dozens of new food ideas. See what is new in the industry and start letting your imagination work for you.

After you have decided just what you want to produce you need to start thinking of some preliminaries. How much is it going to cost to produce? (You need to identify *all* your costs—hidden costs can kill you.) How much can you sell your product for? Spend a day at the supermarket, not as a shopper, but as a market researcher. You can identify how much your competitors are getting for their products, how their packaging sells the products (what works), where your product grouping is located in the store (generic locations, the canned vegetable and fruit aisle, the deli, or the gourmet specialty section), and how to compete for consumer attention within your product area. What shapes work, what catches your eye, what kind of promotions are your competitors using? A day at the supermarket can supply an enormous amount of preliminary market data.

One of the most important things an entrepreneur food processor needs is adequate, accurate information on which to base many of the preliminary decisions concerning the development of a new product. You must have answers to questions such as: Who is going to buy this product? Where does a large population of this consumer group live? How often will this type of product be purchased and in what amounts? What size or amount of this product will be preferred?

Many of these questions can be answered simply by making phone calls and asking. The marketing departments of any major university are a treasure house for this kind of information. Call your local chamber of commerce. Ask them to give you a name of a local manufacturer who is producing a complementary but noncompetitive product. Make an appointment to talk with someone in that organization who handles sales. That person will have a lot of answers for you.

The federal government and most state governments have marketing assistance programs available to small businesses. Refer to Appendices A and B at the end of this volume for additional information.

Marketing research is limited only by your imagination. Much of it you can do with very little cost except your time and mental effort. The key to really effective marketing research is neither technique nor data—it is the amount of actual useful information you are able to gather. Your information must be timely, particularly in the food industry where consumer likes and dislikes are shifting constantly. Once you decide that you are on the right track, go for it!

CHAPTER 2

Developing Your Product

Along with identifying financing, facility and production requirements, and all the hundreds of little details an entrepreneur must deal with during the development stage of the product and the business, it is imperative that the food processor consider several important factors very early on in the research and development stage. These factors are package design, pricing structure, and trademark protection.

Package Design

The design of your product's packaging can mean the success or failure of your product. The packaging is what sells any product to the consumer. Unless the consumer samples the product, which is also a good promotional tool particularly for new products, the only chance you have of convincing a consumer to try your product is through your packaging. When working on your packaging design, take advantage of the enormous display area of new and successful package designs in your supermarket. Walk up and down the aisles and see what catches your attention and why. Color, size, and graphics all are instrumental in creating a successful package.

Keep in mind that, like advertising in magazines or on television, a package or label can impart only as much information as space and your budget allow. Be aware, too, that too "busy" a package will confuse the consumer. Although foil printing, the new "trendy" colors, and four-color process printing are great, are they cost effective for your product? Can you really afford them?

When designing your packaging, keep in mind that federal and state laws and regulations require certain disclosures. (Labeling is discussed in several other sections of the book.) Within the limits of legal requirements, you must decide which information is most important to the consumer and, therefore, deserves greater prominence in packaging and labeling. The Fair Packaging and Labeling Act (FPLA) is the primary federal law requiring mandatory labeling provisions for all consumer goods. The Food and Drug Administration (FDA) has regulatory authority for enforcing the FPLA relative to food.

There are some things to be aware of when developing your package. Prepare packaging and labels that are clear, simple, and to the point. Avoid information "overload" and confusing presentation. Be aware of your responsibilities and of regulations governing packaging and labeling. The following lists suggest several agencies that you can contact for information regarding packaging regulations. Both the federal government and your state government have support staff available to assist small businesses. Your tax dollars pay their salaries, so use them.

Federal Agencies

American National Metric Council, 5410 Grosvenor Lane, Bethesda, MD 20814

Chemical Control Division, Toxic Substances Office, Environmental Protection Agency, Washington, D.C. 20460

Consumer Product Safety Commission, 1111 18th Street, N.W., Washington, D.C. 20036

Federal Trade Commission, Washington, D.C. 20580

Food and Drug Administration, 5600 Fishers Lane, Rockville, MD 20857

National Conference on Weights and Measures, National Bureau of Standards, U.S. Department of Commerce, Washington, D.C. 20234

Office of Metric Programs, U.S. Department of Commerce, Washington, D.C. 20230

State Agencies
The Attorney General of your state, located in the state capitol
The Council of Better Business Bureaus, Inc., 1515 Wilson Boulevard, Arlington, Virginia 22209, or your local Better Business Bureau
The Division of Advertising Practices or the Division of Marketing Practices, Federal Trade Commission, Washington, D.C. 20580
The National Association of Broadcasters, 1771 N Street, N.W., Washington, D.C. 20036
Private counsel or the local Bar Association
State or local Offices of Consumer Protection. Addresses may be obtained from the National Association of Consumer Agency Administrators, 1010 Vermont Avenue, N.W., Suite 1012, Washington, D.C. 20005
U.S. Office of Consumer Affairs, 1009 Premier Building, Washington, D.C. 20201
U.S. Postal Service, Chief Postal Inspector, Washington, D.C. 20260

Be sure to present clear information that identifies the product and the supplier. State the accurate identity of the product by its common or usual name and state the form it takes, for example, garlic paste. Include the name of the manufacturer and who to call if there is a problem or complaint (or compliment). Under U.S. FDA law, all food products and/or labels must display the name, street address, city, state, and zip code of the manufacturer, the packer, or the distributor. The usual name of the food (that which is identified by the average consumer) must appear on the main display panel. The form of the product (e.g., whole, chopped, pitted, pureed, etc.) must be clearly displayed.

You must also state the net quantity of the contents by weight, measure, size, or numerical count. It is wise to indicate the quantity in metric count for potential international sales. The

FDA has strict regulations on these issues. You must state the *net* amount of food in the package. For example, you must use the drained weight when food is packed in liquid that is not consumed as food. If the label identifies contents in number of servings, you must include the size of each serving.

To protect your company name and to ensure your product's integrity, it is important to disclose any change in net volume or net weight of the product and to make sure it is prominently presented on your packaging. A change in volume occurs naturally when a product "settles," as with most cereals. A statement such as the following will provide reassuring information to the buyer regarding this condition: "This package is sold by weight, not by volume. It contains full net weight indicated. If it does not appear full when opened, it is because contents have settled during shipping and handling."

It is extremely important to notify the consumer through package promotion when the net weight is adjusted. Minor net-weight reduction is often used to retain the same retail price. Remember when many of our favorite chocolate bars seemed to be shrinking before our eyes? This reduction was necessary at the time to counter rising cocoa and sugar prices. The major chocolate manufacturers opted for a reduction in product weight rather than an increase in product cost. Those manufacturers who were honest with consumers identified net-weight reduction and this explains why they have maintained their market shares. Those few who didn't have suffered. Surveys of complaint data show that consumers are resentful and often change buying preferences when price increases are avoided by making unannounced reductions in net product weight.

Disclose truthful information about the ingredients in the product. (Remember the Beech-Nut baby food boys? If not, see Chapter 6.) Federal and state laws require that food packaging clearly identify nutrient value, salt and sugar content, calories, minimum daily requirements per serving of vitamins, protein, carbohydrates, and fat, and recommended serving size on which the nutrient value is calculated.

Make sure that price information is clearly displayed, particularly if part of your market thrust is price competition. The advent of UPC codes and product price scanners in many of the larger grocery stores has eliminated some of the past effectiveness of this strategy. If your product falls into a specialty food niche, this information should be considered essential.

In the early 1970s, with the rapid development of computer technology, the food industry began to experiment with a new method of inventory control called the UPC system. The UPC system consists of the universal product bar code (Box 2.1) and an electronic scanning device. The system was developed by the food industry to give every product a unique code number. This number allows simpler and more accurate product identification. The symbol makes possible the use of scanner-equipped checkstands which speed customer checkout operations, reduce item price-marking requirements, and enable the retailer to collect complete and accurate information on all aspects of sales transactions. Most likely, within 3–5 years the major retailers will require UPC coding on every product they sell.

It would be wise to include a UPC in your packaging designs. It will save you time and money when a retailer who requires UPCs decides to shelf your product.

For more information on the UPC System contact:

> Uniform Code Council, Inc.
> 8163 Old Yankee Rd., Suite J
> Dayton, OH 45458
> (513) 435-3870

The Uniform Code Council is the central management and information center for manufacturers and retailers participating in the system. This organization is not a government agency. It is an administrative council which exists specifically to control the issuing of codes, to provide detailed information, and to coordinate the efforts of all participants. Although membership in the Uniform Code Council is voluntary, it is required to

BOX 2.1

= 012345-67890:
(Note: First 6 digits
assigned by UCC,
Inc.; second 5 by
manufacturer); 12th
is a check digit.

The universal product code (UPC) is a 12-digit, all-numeric code that will identify the consumer package. The code consists of a number-system character, a 5-digit manufacturer identification number, and a 5-digit item code number.

Number System Character. The first position in the 11-digit UPC code, the number-system character serves to "key" the other numbers as to meaning as well as category. There are currently seven categories of the number-system character:

0 Assigned to all items *except* as follows:

2 Assigned to random-weight items such as meat and produce

3 Assigned to companies which have been delegated their NDC number as their UPC

4 Assigned for retailer use only

5 Assigned to coupons

6 and 7 Assigned to industrial applications as well as retail applications, where they serve the same function as 0.

Manufacturer Identification Number. The manufacturer identification number is a 5-digit number assigned by Uniform Code Council, Inc.

Item Code Number. The item code is a 5-digit number assigned and controlled by the member company. The item code should be unique for each consumer package and/or shipping container.

The 12-digit universal product code plus a scanner-readable check digit are represented in the bars and spaces that make up the complete scanner-readable symbol. The check digit enables the scanner system to immediately verify the accurate data translation of the universal product code as the symbol is scanned.

obtain a manufacturer's number assignment (see Fig. 2.1). Cost of membership is based on sales volume.

The Council was originally created by several grocery industry associations. Council membership has expanded to include drug, discount, and department stores, non-food manufacturers, wholesalers, and distributors, as well as companies from the wine and alcoholic beverage industries. The Council has a full-time staff to help you.

Remember, your product packaging is your greatest promotional vehicle; for example, give prominence to facts pertinent to the consumer's purchasing decision. Priority information includes price, contents and ingredients, instructions for use and preparation, storage and shelf life, packaging date, and terms and conditions of promotional premiums (e.g., coupons, "free" gifts, etc.).

Design your package right the first time. Take into consideration all the features necessary to protect the quality and form of the contents during distribution, shelf life, and storage.

Whenever possible, design packaging with easy access to the contents and, when appropriate, provide an economical and effective means for resealing the package. Convenience has become as important a factor in consumer appeal as price. Many of the larger grocery chains are insisting on some kind of tamper-proof packaging (e.g., safety seals, vacuum buttons, bottle-cap collars, etc.).

If you feel that your product may have potential overseas market appeal, it would be wise to design your packaging for export shipments. You will save yourself a lot of time and money if your packaging is adaptable enough to meet other countries' requirements. Another advantage to properly designed "universal" packaging is that you don't lose precious lead time in supplying product to interested foreign buyers while you are trying to repackage your product.

For several of the larger overseas markets, the minor addition of the U.S.A. manufacturer's address and metric weight classification can make your product's packaging "universal." Even in Canada, where the bilingualization regulations are exceptionally strict, you can usually "launch" your product to test consumer

Application for Universal Product Code and Uniform Code Council, Inc. Membership**

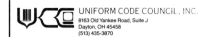

UNIFORM CODE COUNCIL, INC.
8163 Old Yankee Road, Suite J
Dayton, OH 45458
(513) 435-3870

(Note: Failure to complete the form in full will result in a delay in processing.)

Company Name
(When entering "Company Name" do NOT use "dba's," brand names, or product names. Enter the name under which your company is registered to do business.)

Name of Parent Company

Street (necessary for UPS delivery of package)

Name(s) of your Subsidiary

City   State   Zip

P.O. Box and Zip

Name of Chief Executive Officer   Title   ( ) Phone

Name of Key Contact for UPC   Title   ( ) Phone

"Name of Key Contact for UPC" should be the individual within your company who will be assigning your UPC item numbers and to whom any questions or correspondence regarding your UPC program should be addressed. Please do not provide the name of your printer, film master supplier or advertising agency.

TYPE OF COMPANY: (please check one)

☐ Manufacturer ☐ Retailer*   ☐ Foodservice   ☐ Wholesale   ☐ Importer
                                        Distributor*   Distributor*

☐ Wholesaler* ☐ Other (describe)_____   ☐ Broker*   ☐ Buying Group* ☐ Jobber

*If a retailer, wholesaler, wholesale distributor, foodservice distributor, broker, or buying group does not have its own private label products, a UPC manufacturer identification number is not required and will not be assigned. If the organization does have its own private label products, the UPC fee is based upon the annual sales of the private label products only.

MAJOR PRODUCT CATEGORY

Provide general type of product marketed by your company (i.e., frozen food, hosiery, apparel, hardware, etc.)

Does your company have a National Drug Code (NDC) number?_____ Number _____

If available, do you wish to have this number assigned as your UPC number? _____

The membership fee is based on latest annual U.S. domestic $ sales volume in (1) retail stores including supermarkets, drug, mass merchandise/discount, hardware, liquor, military commissaries, military exchanges and department stores; and (2) through institutional and foodservice channels (e.g., restaurants, hotels, hospitals, schools). In addition, the fee is based on *total U.S. domestic retail dollar sales volume of your company,* not just on the products which you choose to code at this time. If you provide your products to distributors/wholesalers who then sell to the retail trade, you must provide your best estimate as to the actual retail dollar sales volume which results.

Retailers: (should be used **only if you own and operate actual retail outlets** (i.e., supermarkets, discount stores, hardware stores, retail liquor stores, drug stores, etc.).	**Manufacturers, Importers, Buying Groups, Brokers, Jobbers, Wholesalers, Foodservice Distributors, Wholesale/Distributors**
	$0 to $1.550 Million $300
	$1.550 to $10 Million . . . . $200 per million $ of sales
Under $60 Million $300	(parts of millions rounded to
$60-$99 Million $500	nearest $100,000)
$100 Million to $1 Billion $1,000	$10-$99 Million . . . . $2,000 flat fee
$1 Billion to $5 Billion $2,500	$100-$499 Million . . . . $6,000 flat fee
Over $5 Billion $5,000	$500 Million and Over . . . . $10,000 flat fee

Specific Annual Sales $_____   Fee $_____   (add $50 if company applying for membership
**The Uniform Code Council, Inc. is a non-profit membership organization.   is located outside the United States or Canada)
(continued on second side of form)

Figure 2.1 Application for Universal Product Code and Universal Code Council, Inc. membership. (*continues*)

Guidelines for the use of the UPC and symbol and your UPC manufacturer identification number* (if applicable) will be sent to you on receipt of your check and Council approval of your completed application. Membership includes one set of all current UPC manuals.

All reasonable precautions have been taken to prevent the assignment of duplicate UPC manufacturer identification numbers. If duplicate numbers are assigned, the liability of the Council shall be limited to a refund of the applicant's membership fee.

*The system is designed to provide *one* UPC manufacturer identification number to each member. In special circumstances, a member may require more than one identification number. If you believe this is necessary in your company, please write separately to Uniform Code Council, Inc., 8163 Old Yankee Road, Suite J, Dayton, Ohio 45458.

OUR COMPANY HEREBY APPLIES FOR MEMBERSHIP IN THE UNIFORM CODE COUNCIL, INC.
A CHECK COVERING OUR MEMBERSHIP FEE IS ENCLOSED.

_____   _____   _____
Signature   Title   Date

MAILING THE FORM AND MEMBERSHIP FEE TO THE UC COUNCIL

If returning your form and fee via regular first class mail, send it to P.O. Box 1244, Dayton, OH 45401-1244. DO NOT SEND TO THE STREET ADDRESS.

If returning your form and fee via U.S. Postal Service Express Mail or by some form of courier (i.e., Federal Express, DHL, etc.), send to 8163 Old Yankee Rd., Suite J, Dayton, OH 45458 NOT TO THE P.O. BOX.

RETURN OF YOUR UPC NUMBER BY THE UC COUNCIL

The Council will **not** provide the assigned UPC number by telephone or FAX.

If you are located in the U.S., allow 7-10 working days for return of the UPC number by United Parcel Service. Packages addressed outside the U.S. will be sent via 1st class mail.

PRIORITY HANDLING INSTRUCTIONS

If your intent is to ask the Council for a quicker turnaround time, priority charges will apply and **must be included with the application and membership fee.** We will be unable to accommodate such a request once the application has been received, should such priority charges not be included. **We will not return packages COD.**

If you are located in the U.S., the Council uses **only** United Parcel Service as the courier for overnight return of UPC numbers. You must include priority handling charges and prepayment of the UPS next day charges as follows: $34.25 if located within the 48 contiguous states, $36.25 if in Alaska or Hawaii and $38.50 if in Puerto Rico.

If you are located outside the U.S., the package will be shipped via DHL. You must include an additional $75 for priority handling and prepayment of DHL charges. If you include the priority handling and UPS Next Day Air/ DHL charges **DO NOT SEND YOUR APPLICATION TO THE P.O. BOX.** The result would be a delay of one day in the return of your UPC number and technical manuals. Send it to 8163 Old Yankee Rd., Suite J, Dayton, OH 45458.

Return completed application form and check to: Uniform Code Council, Inc.
P.O. Box 1244
Dayton, Ohio 45401-1244

For additional information contact: Uniform Code Council, Inc.
(513) 435-3870

Figure 2.1 (*continued*)

acceptance if these two additions are included. The bilingualization problem is addressed in greater detail in Chapter 8.

Trademarks

After you have put considerable time, effort, and money into designing your product and package, you need to make sure you protect your work. One of the easiest and most effective ways for the food processor to do this is by registering his or her trademark.

A trademark is a word, name, or symbol used to identify your product and to distinguish it from those being sold by other companies. It indicates who made the product and, if you've done your job, it will indicate the guaranteed quality of any items bearing your mark.

New food processors are often confused by the difference between a trademark and a trade name. A trademark identifies *the source of* product, while a trade name *is the name under which* the producer *is doing business.* If you plan on selling your product strictly within the borders of your state, you need only register your trademark in your state, usually through your Secretary of State's office. If you plan on selling your product in other states as well, you will need to register your trademark through

> The U.S. Department of Commerce
> Patent and Trademark Office
> Washington, D.C. 20031
> (703) 557-3883 or 557-3881

The rights of a trademark are established when the work, name, or symbol is used in commerce. In 1989, Congress passed a law that brought the United States in line with the rest of the world in recognizing the registration of trademarks with an "intent to use" rather than requiring actual use. Thus, a business person who has an idea for the name of a product or company or service can register that name and subsequently provide evidence of actual use to finalize the registration. One result of this is that people may register names which they are not actually using. This makes it harder for an individual to be sure that he is not using a name already claimed by someone else, but it also highlights the need for a reasonably careful search by an entrepreneur before he begins using a name as follows:

(1) Search trade publications and directories along with any other logical (nonlegal) sources to be sure that the name that has been chosen is not already in use for food products or services. If starting out on a large scale, the entrepreneur may wish to pay for a more formal trademark search to be conducted. This can be done through a variety of services or commissioned by an attorney. The cost is approximately $500.

(2) If you wish to seek formal trademark protection, application for registration of a trademark may be made based on an intent to use the name. You will obtain registration for six months which can extended for additional six-month periods up to a total of 24 months. There are fees involved with this. When you begin using the name, simply supply the specimens to the U.S. Patent and Trademark Office which finalizes the registration. This is, of course, something you should obtain legal advice on.

(3) As an additional resource, contact the U.S. Trademark Association which is located at 6 East 45th Street, New York, NY 10017. The telephone number if (212) 986-5880.

Besides the written application (see Fig. 2.2), you must submit a drawing of mark, five specimens or facsimiles of the actual product mark, and a filing fee. Trademarks registered with the federal government are valid for 20 years and may be renewed for additional 20-year terms if the mark is still used in interstate commerce.

The following information is taken directly from a publication by the U.S. Department of Commerce Patent and Trade Office.

TRADEMARK/SERVICE MARK APPLICATION, PRINCIPAL REGISTER, WITH DECLARATION	MARK (Identify the mark)
	CLASS NO. (If known)

TO THE ASSISTANT SECRETARY AND COMMISSIONER OF PATENTS AND TRADEMARKS:

APPLICANT NAME:

APPLICANT BUSINESS ADDRESS:

APPLICANT ENTITY: (Check one and supply requested information)

☐ Individual - Citizenship: (Country) _____

☐ Partnership - Partnership Domicile: (State and Country) _____
Names and Citizenship (Country) of General Partners: _____
_____

☐ Corporation - State (Country, if appropriate) of Incorporation: _____

☐ Other: (Specify Nature of Entity and Domicile) _____
_____

GOODS AND/OR SERVICES:

Applicant requests registration of the above-identified trademark/service mark shown in the accompanying drawing in the United States Patent and Trademark Office on the Principal Register established by the Act of July 5, 1946 (15 U.S.C. 1051 et. seq., as amended.) for the following goods/services: _____
_____

BASIS FOR APPLICATION: (Check one or more, but NOT both the first AND second boxes, and supply requested information)

☐ Applicant is using the mark in commerce on or in connection with the above identified goods/services. (15 U.S.C. 1051(a), as amended.) Three specimens showing the mark as used in commerce are submitted with this application.
- Date of first use of the mark anywhere: _____
- Date of first use of the mark in commerce which the U.S. Congress may regulate:_____
- Specify the type of commerce: _____
(e.g., interstate, between the U.S. and a specified foreign country)
- Specify manner or mode of use of mark on or in connection with the goods/services:_____
_____
(e.g., trademark is applied to labels, service mark is used in advertisements)

☐ Applicant has a bona fide intention to use the mark in commerce on or in connection with the above identified goods/services. (15 U.S.C. 1051(b), as amended.)
- Specify intended manner or mode of use of mark on or in connection with the goods/services:_____
_____
(e.g., trademark will be applied to labels, service mark will be used in advertisements)

☐ Applicant has a bona fide intention to use the mark in commerce on or in connection with the above identified goods/services, and asserts a claim of priority based upon a foreign application in accordance with 15 U.S.C. 1126(d), as amended.
- Country of foreign filing: _____ • Date of foreign filing: _____

☐ Applicant has a bona fide intention to use the mark in commerce on or in connection with the above identified goods/services and, accompanying this application, submits a certification or certified copy of a foreign registration in accordance with 15 U.S.C. 1126(e), as amended.
- Country of registration:_____ • Registration number: _____

Note: Declaration, on Reverse Side, MUST be Signed

PTO Form 1478 (REV. 9/89)
OMB No. 06510009
Exp. 5-31-91

U.S. DEPARTMENT OF COMMERCE/Patent and Trademark Office

Figure 2.2 Trademark and Service Mark Application, Principal Register, with Declaration (*continues*).

DECLARATION

The undersigned being hereby warned that willful false statements and the like so made are punishable by fine or imprisonment, or both, under 18 U.S.C. 1001, and that such willful false statements may jeopardize the validity of the application or any resulting registration, declares that he/she is properly authorized to execute this application on behalf of the applicant; he/she believes the applicant to be the owner of the trademark/service mark sought to be registered, or, if the application is being filed under 15 U.S.C. 1051(b), he/she believes applicant to be entitled to use such mark in commerce; to the best of his/her knowledge and belief no other person, firm, corporation, or association has the right to use the above identified mark in commerce, either in the identical form thereof or in such near resemblance thereto as to be likely, when used on or in connection with the goods/services of such other person, to cause confusion, or to cause mistake, or to deceive; and that all statements made of his/her own knowledge are true and all statements made on information and belief are believed to be true.

_____
Date

_____
Signature

_____
Telephone Number

_____
Print or Type Name and Position

INSTRUCTIONS AND INFORMATION FOR APPLICANT

To receive a filing date, the application must be completed and **signed by the applicant** and submitted along with:

1. The prescribed fee for each class of goods/services listed in the application;
2. A drawing of the mark in conformance with 37 CFR 2.52;
3. If the application is based on use of the mark in commerce, three (3) specimens (evidence) of the mark as used in commerce for each class of goods/services listed in the application. All three specimens may be the same and may be in the nature of: (a) labels showing the mark which are placed on the goods; (b) a photograph of the mark as it appears on the goods, (c) brochures or advertisements showing the mark as used in connection with the services.

Verification of the application - The application must be signed in order for the application to receive a filing date. Only the following person may sign the verification (Declaration) for the application, depending on the applicant's legal entity: (1) the individual applicant; (b) an officer of the corporate applicant; (c) one general partner of a partnership applicant; (d) all joint applicants.

Additional information concerning the requirements for filing an application are available in a booklet entitled **Basic Facts about Trademarks,** which may be obtained by writing:

U.S. DEPARTMENT OF COMMERCE
Patent and Trademark Office
Washington, D.C. 20231

Or by calling: (703) 557-INFO

This form is estimated to take 15 minutes to complete. Time will vary depending upon the needs of the individual case. Any comments on the amount of time you require to complete this form should be sent to the Office of Management and Organization, U.S. Patent and Trademark Office, U.S. Department of Commerce, Washington D.C., 20231, and to the Office of Information and Regulatory Affairs, Office of Management and Budget, Washington, D.C. 20503.

Figure 2.2 *(continued).*

Benefits of Registration

While federal registration is not necessary for trademark protection, registration on the Principal Register does provide certain advantages:

1. The filing date of the application is a constructive date of first use of the mark in commerce (this gives registrant nationwide priority as of that date, except as to certain prior users or prior applicants);
2. The right to sue in federal court for trademark infringement;
3. Recovery of profits, damages and costs in a federal court infringement action and the possibility of treble damages and attorneys' fees;
4. Constructive notice of a claim of ownership (which eliminates a good faith defense for a party adopting the trademark subsequent to the registrant's date of registration);
5. The right to deposit the registration with Customs in order to stop the importation of goods bearing an infringing mark;
6. Prima facie evidence of the validity of the registration, registrant's ownership of the mark and of registrant's exclusive right to use the mark in commerce in connection with the goods or services specified in the certificate;
7. The possibility of incontestability, in which case the registration constitutes conclusive evidence of the registrant's exclusive right, with certain limited exceptions, to use the registered mark in commerce;
8. Limited grounds for attacking a registration once it is five years old;
9. Availability of criminal penalties and treble damages in an action for counterfeiting a registered trademark;
10. A basis for filing trademark applications in foreign countries.

Notice

Once a Federal registration is issued, the registrant may give notice of registration by using the ® symbol, or the phrase "Registered in U.S. Patent and Trademark Office" or "Reg. U.S. Pat. & Tm. Off." Although registration symbols may not be lawfully used prior to registration, many trademark owners use a TM or SM (if the mark identifies a service) symbol to indicate a claim of ownership, even if no federal trademark application is pending.

The Registration Process

The Patent and Trademark Office (PTO) is responsible for the federal registration of trademarks. When an application is filed, it is reviewed to determine if it meets the requirements for receiving a filing date. If the filing requirements are not met, the entire mailing, including the fee, is returned to the applicant. If the application meets the filing requirements, it is assigned a serial number, and the applicant is sent a filing receipt.

The first part of the registration process is a determination by the trademark examining attorney as to whether the mark may be registered. An initial determination of registrability, listing any statutory grounds for refusal as well as any procedural informalities in the application, is issued about three months after filing. The applicant must respond to any objections raised within six months, or the application will be considered abandoned. If, after reviewing the applicant's response, the examining attorney makes a final refusal of registration, the applicant may appeal to the Trademark Trial and Appeal Board, an administrative tribunal within the PTO.

Once the examining attorney approves the mark, the mark will be published in the *Trademark Official Gazette*, a weekly publication of the PTO. Any other party then has 30 days to oppose the registration of the mark, or request an extension of time to oppose. An opposition is similar to a proceeding in the Federal district courts, but is held before the Trademark Trial and Appeal Board. If no opposition is filed, the application enters the next stage of the registration process.

If the mark is published based upon its actual use in commerce, registration will be issued approximately 12 weeks from the date the mark was published.

If, instead, the mark published based upon applicant's statement of a bona fide intention to use the mark in commerce, a *notice of allowance* will issue approximately 12 weeks from the date the mark was published. The applicant then has six months from the date of the notice of allowance to either (1) use the mark in commerce and submit a *statement of use*, or (2) request a six-month *extension of time* to file a statement of use (see forms and instructions at back of booklet). The applicant may request additional extensions of time only as noted in the instructions on the back of the form.

Statutory Grounds For Refusal

The examining attorney will refuse registration if the mark or term applied for:

1. Does not function as a trademark to identify the goods or services as coming from a particular source; for example, the matter applied for is merely ornamentation;
2. Is immoral, deceptive or scandalous;
3. May disparage or falsely suggest a connection with persons, institutions, beliefs or national symbols, or bring them into contempt or disrepute;
4. Consists of or simulates the flag or coat of arms or other insignia of the United States, or a state or municipality, or any foreign nation;
5. Is the name, portrait or signature of a particular living individual, unless he has given written consent; or is the name, signature or portrait of a deceased president of the United States during the life of his widow, unless she has given her consent;
6. So resembles a mark already registered in the PTO as to be likely, when used on or in connection with the goods of the applicant, to cause confusion, or to cause mistake, or to deceive;
7. Is merely descriptive or deceptively misdescriptive of the goods or services;
8. Is primarily geographically descriptive or deceptively misdescriptive of the goods or services of the applicant;
9. Is primarily merely a surname.

A mark will not be refused registration on the grounds listed in numbers 7, 8 and 9 if the applicant can show that, through use of the mark in commerce, the mark has become distinctive so that it now identifies to the public the applicant's goods or services. Marks which are refused registration on the grounds listed in numbers 1, 7, 8 and 9 may be registrable on the *Supplemental Register*, which contains terms or designs considered capable of distinguishing the owner's goods or services, but that do not yet do so. A term or design cannot be considered for registration on the *Supplemental Register* unless it is in use in commerce in relation to all the goods or services identified in the application, and an acceptable allegation of use has been submitted. If a mark is registered on the *Supplemental Register*, the registrant may bring suit for trademark infringement in the federal courts, or may use the registration as a basis for filing in some foreign countries. None of the other benefits of federal registration listed on page 1 apply. An applicant may file an application on the *Principal Register* and, if appropriate, amend the application to the *Supplemental Register* for no additional fee.

Trademark Search Library

A record of all active registrations and pending applications is maintained by the PTO to help determine whether a previously registered mark exists which could prevent the registration of an applicant's mark. (See ground for refusal No. 6, above.) The search library is located near Washington, D.C. at Crystal Plaza 2, 2nd Floor, 2011 Jefferson Davis Highway, Arlington, VA 22022, and is open to the public free of charge Monday through Friday, 8:00 am to 5:30 pm. The PTO cannot advice prospective applicants of the availability of a particular mark prior to the filing of an application. The applicant may hire a private search company or law firm to perform a search if a search is desired before filing an application and the applicant is unable to visit the search library. The PTO cannot recommend any such companies, but the applicant may wish to consult listings for "Trademark Search Services" in the telephone directories or contact local bar associations for a list of attorneys specializing in trademark law.

Who May File an Application

The owners of marks may file and prosecute their own applications for registration, or be represented by an attorney. The PTO cannot help select an attorney.

Filing Requirements

An application consists of (1) a written application form; (2) a drawing of the mark; (3) three specimens showing actual use of the mark on or in connection with the goods or services, (4) the required filing fee; and, *only if the application is filed based upon prior use of the mark in commerce.* A separate application must be filed for each mark for which registration is requested.

Following is a description of each of these elements of a complete application. The written application form is the first form of four forms at the back of the booklet and is titled "Trademark/Service" Mark Application, Principal Register, with Declaration."

1. Written Application Form

The application must be written in English. The enclosed form may be used for either a trademark or service mark application. Additional forms may be photocopied. The following explanation covers each blank, beginning at the top.

Heading. Identify (a) the mark (e.g. "ERGO" or "ERGO and design") and (b) the class number(s) of the goods or services for which registration is sought. Classification is part of the PTO's administrative processing. The international classification of goods and services is used (see inside back cover of this booklet). The class may be left blank if the appropriate class number is not known.

Applicant. The application must be filed in the name of the owner of the mark. Specify, if an individual, applicant's name and citizenship; if a partnership, the names and citizenship of the general partners and the domicile of the partnership; if a corporation or association, the name under which it is incorporated and the state or foreign nation under the laws of which it is organized. Also indicate the applicant's post office address.

Identification of Goods or Services. State briefly the specific goods or services for which the mark is used or intended to be used and for which registration is sought. Use clear and precise language, for example, "women's clothing namely, blouses and skirts," or "computer programs for use by accountants," or "retail food store services." Note that the identification of goods or services should describe the goods the applicant sells or the services the applicant renders, not the medium in which the mark appears, which is often advertising. "Advertising" in this context identifies a service rendered by advertising agencies. For example, a restaurateur would identify his service as "restaurant services," not "menus, signs, etc." which is the medium through which the mark is communicated.

Basis for Application. The applicant must check at least one of four boxes to specify the basis for filing the application. Usually an application is based upon either (1) prior use of the mark in commerce (the first box), or (2) a bona fide intention to use the mark in commerce (the second box), but not both. If both the first and second boxes are checked, the Patent and Trademark Office will *not* accept the application and will return it to the applicant without processing.

The last two boxes pertain to applications filed in the United States pursuant to international agreements, based upon applications or registrations in foreign countries. These bases are asserted relatively infrequently. For further information about foreign-based applications, the applicant may call the trademark information number listed in this booklet or contact a private attorney.

If the applicant is using the mark in commerce in relation to all the goods or services listed in the application, check the first box and state each of the following:

- The date the trademark was first used anywhere in the United States on the goods, or in connection with the services, specified in the application;
- The date the trademark was first used on the specified goods, or in connection with the specified services, sold or shipped (or rendered) in a type of commerce which may be regulated by Congress;

- The type of commerce in which the goods were sold or shipped or services were rendered [for example, "interstate commerce" or "commerce between the United States and (specify foreign country)"]; and
- How the mark is used on the goods, or in connection with the services [for example, "the mark is used on labels which are affixed to the goods," or "the mark is used in advertisements for the services"].

If the applicant has a bona fide intention to use the mark in commerce in relation to the goods or services specified in the application, check the second box. This would include situations where the mark has not been used at all or where the mark has been used on the specified goods or services only within a single state (intrastate commerce).

Execution. The application form must be dated and signed. (See back of form.) The declaration and signature block appear on the back of the form. The PTO will *not* accept an unsigned application and will return it to the applicant without processing. By signing the form, the applicant is swearing that all the information in the application is believed to be true. If the applicant is an individual, the individual must execute it; if joint applicants, all must execute; if a partnership, one general partner must execute the application; and if a corporation or association, one officer of the organization must execute the application.

2. Drawing

The drawing is a representation of the mark as actually used or intended to be used on the goods or services. There are two types; (a) typed drawings and (b) special form drawings. All drawings must be on pure white, durable, nonshiny paper in 8½ in. wide by 11 in. long. One of the shorter sides of the sheet should be regarded as its top. There must be a margin of at least one inch on the sides and bottom of the paper and at least one inch between the drawing of the mark and the heading.

The *drawing* is different than the *specimens*, which are the actual tags or labels (for goods) or advertisements (for services) which evidence use of the mark in commerce. The *drawing* is a black and white, or typed, rendition of the mark which is used in printing the mark in the *Official Gazette* and on the registration certificate. A copy of the drawing is also filed in the paper records of the trademark search library to provide notice of the pending application.

The heading runs across the top of the drawing, beginning one inch from the top edge and not exceeding one third of the sheet; on separate lines list the following:

- Applicant's name;
- Applicant's post office address;
- The goods or services specified in the application (or typical items of the goods or services if there are many goods or services listed);
- Only in an application based on use in commerce—the date of first use of the mark anywhere in the United States and the date of first use of the mark in commerce;
- Only in an application based on a foriegn application—the filing date of the foreign application.

Typed drawing. If the mark is only words, or words and numerals, and the applicant does not wish the registration to be issued for a particular depiction of the words and numerals, the mark may be typed in capital letters in the center of the page.

Special form drawing. This form must be used if the applicant wishes the registration for the mark to be issued in a particular style, or if the mark contains a design element. The drawing of the mark must be done in black ink, either with an india ink pen or by a process which will give satisfactory reproduction characteristics. Every line and letter, including words, must be black. This applies to all lines, including lines used for shading. Half-tones and gray are not acceptable. All lines must be clean, sharp, and solid, and not be fine or crowded. A photolithographic reproduction, printer's proof or camera ready copy may be used if otherwise suitable. Photographs are not acceptable. Photocopies are acceptable only if they produce an unusually clear and sharp black and white rendering. The use of white pigment to cover lines is not acceptable.

The preferred size of the drawing of the mark is 2½ in. × 2½ in., and in no case may it be larger than 4 in. × 4 in. The Patent and Trademark Office will not accept an application with a special form drawing depicted larger than 4 in. by 4 in. and will return the application without processing. If the amount of detail in the mark precludes clear reduction to the required 4 in. × 4 in. size, such detail should not be shown in the drawing but should be verbally described in the body of the application.

Where color is a feature of a mark, the color or colors may be designated in the drawing by the linings shown in Figure 2.3

3. Specimens (Examples of Use)

Trademarks may be placed on the goods; on the container for the goods; on displays associated with the goods; on tags or labels attached to the goods; or, if the nature of the goods makes such placement impractical, then on documents associated with the goods or their sale. Service marks may appear in advertisements for the services, or in brochures about the services, or on business cards or stationary used in connection with the services.

For an application based on actual use of the mark in commerce, the applicant must furnish three examples of use, as described in the paragraph above, when the application is filed. The PTO will not accept an application based on use in commerce without at least one "specimen" and will return it to the applicant without processing.

The three "specimens" may be identical or they may be examples of three different types of uses. The three specimens should be actual labels, tags, containers, or displays for goods; and actual advertisements, brochures, store signs, or stationary (if

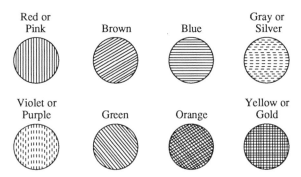

Figure 2.3 Color Designations in Trademark Drawings.

the nature of the services is clear from the letterhead or body of the letter) for services. Specimens may not be larger than 8½ in. by 11 in. and must be capable of being arranged flat. Three-dimensional or bulky material is not acceptable. Photographs or other reproductions clearly and legibly showing the mark on the goods, or on displays associated with the goods, may be submitted if the manner of affixing the mark to the goods, or the nature of the goods, is such that specimens as described above cannot be submitted.

4. Filing Fee

The fee, effective April 17, 1989, is $175 for each class of goods or services for which the application is made. At least $175 must be submitted for the application to be given a filing date. All payments should be made in United States specie, treasury notes, national bank notes, post office money orders, or certified checks. Personal or business checks may be submitted. The PTO will cancel credit if payment cannot be collected. Money orders and checks should be made payable to the Commissioner of Patents and Trademarks. Money sent by mail to the PTO will be at the risk of the sender; letters containing cash should be registered. Remittances made from foreign countries must be payable and immediately negotiable in the United States for the full amount of the fee required. Application fees are non-refundable.

Further Requirements for Intent-to-Use Applicants

An applicant who alleges only a bona fide intention to use a mark in commerce must make use of the mark in commerce before a registration will be issued. After use begins, the applicant must submit, along with specimens evidencing use and a fee of $100 per class of goods or services in the application, either (1) an Amendment to Allege Use or (2) a Statement of Use. The difference between the two filings is the timing of the filing. Copies of each of these forms appear in the back of this booklet behind the application form. See the instructions and information concerning the filing of these forms on the back of each form.

Also in the back of this booklet is a form entitled "Request for Extension of Time under 37 CFR 2.89 to File a Statement of Use, with Declaration." This form is intended for use only when an applicant needs to request an extension of time to file a statement of use. See the instructions and information concerning the use of this form on the back of the form.

Foreign Applicants

Domestic Representative. Applicants not living in the United States must designate by a written document the name and address of some person resident in the United States on whom notices of process in proceedings affecting the mark may be served. This person will also receive all official communications unless the applicant is represented by an attorney in the United States.

Communications with the PTO

The application and all other communications should be addressed to "The Commissioner of Patents and Trademarks, Washington, D.C., 20231." It is preferred that the applicant indicate its telephone number on the application, form. Once a serial number is assigned to the application, the applicant should refer to this number in all telephone and written communications concerning the application.

Additional Information

The Federal registration of trademarks is governed by the Trademark Act of 1946, 15 U.S.C. Sec. 1051 *et seq.*; the Rules, 37 C.F.R. Part 2; and the Trademark Manual of Examining Procedure.

- General Trademark or Patent Information: (703) 557-INFO
- Status Information for Particular Trademark Applications: (703) 557-5249
- General Copyright Information: (202) 479-0700

Pricing

There are some general principles to follow when you are pricing your product. The initial price of a new product, that is the price at launch, is one of the most important elements of your marketing strategies, yet it is often given the least amount of careful consideration. An overpriced product with no other marketable features will gather dust quickly on a grocer's shelf, or an underpriced product will bankrupt you.

There are some very basic concepts to follow when establishing your pricing. A golden rule to remember is "the higher the price of your product, in comparison to your competition, the fewer units you will sell." Lowering prices is not always your best option.

As a rule, as a small food manufacturer you should not plan on competing on the basis of price alone unless some element of your production procedure allows you to compete on a low-cost level. In other words, if you are producing garlic paste and you happen to grow your own garlic on a large farm in a rural area where there is an unlimited labor force available to you at minimum wage, and you just happen to own the building where you are processing the product, you probably could undercut your competition. On the other hand, if you are producing a quality salsa but sourcing your raw materials and packaging in relatively small volumes from local brokers, you wouldn't want to try to compete with the pricing of Pace Picante Sauce.

You should compete on the basis of product quality, uniqueness, delivery time, or whatever advantage you can offer customers over your competitors. There are many things to take into consideration when determining a price for your product. Along with internal costs (what it costs to produce your product) you must also take into consideration market factors, the economy, technology competition, and resources. Keep in mind that it is the market, much more than your actual costs, that determines the price at which your product will sell. Only if you can sell your product at a price somewhere between your cost plus your desired profit and the price the market has set can you hope to be successful. I am constantly amazed at the number of small food manufacturers who don't know what it costs them to produce their products. Too often, the new food processor is producing a product without specifically tracking all internal costs. This is a *huge* mistake and could easily prove catastrophic for a new business. Good management of all aspects of your company depends on good information. This is just as true for pricing as it is for understanding the operating aspects of a small food processing business. If you don't have accurate figures, find a good accountant to develop them for you, and fast! Once you have reliable basic cost data, you can figure your cost plus profit and your price. When you have established your cost-plus-profit figure, your next step is to identify a "price ceiling." A price ceiling is that particular price established in your market for a particular item. Two approaches can be used to determine the price ceiling. They are "hit or miss" and market research.

The hit-or-miss approach requires that the product be produced, priced, and put on the market with a "trial by fire" attitude toward pricing. A very important principle of consumer psychology is that it is much easier to accept lowered prices than raised prices. Consequently, it is better to put a new product on the market with an extra margin built in for possible price reduction. If the market accepts the price with the extra margin included, more rapid recovery of costs will occur. If the price is not accepted, it can be reduced to stimulate sales. Obviously, this method is riskier and potentially more damaging to a start-up business than one which investigates the market prior to establishing product price.

The market research approach eliminates the risk of determining what price the market will bear after a product is placed on the shelf. Most new food processors don't use this method in an attempt to avoid the inevitable added expense of consulting marketing experts. The choice between hit-or-miss and market research should be based on a comparison of the cost of manufacturing and test marketing a small quantity of the product and the cost of obtaining market research data. You might hire an independent processor to manufacture your product in small quantities in order to test the market *before* you invest in your own production facility.

Many small food manufacturers choose not to use outside marketing research support to help establish their price and particular market niche. In many ways this seems to be a classic case of "pound wise and penny foolish." Starting a food processing business is not cheap. The capital required for equipment, raw materials, supplies, facility acquisition, labor, etc., is enormous. Granted, marketing consultants are usually expensive, but if you wisely focus your efforts, the full cost of a marketing study should be a fraction of your first year's expenses and will save you many dollars in the long run. A big part of the expense that you will be charged will be for trade numbers (industry statistics for your particular product). The consultant obtains these numbers from one of the national market research companies (i.e., Nielsen or TMIC). If you feel this type of data is all the information you will need to strategize your own marketing plan, then why not go directly to one of these companies? The following is a list of a few of the research companies that can provide you with trade numbers.

1. Nielson
   707 Lake Cook Road
   Deerfield, IL 60015
   (312) 480-6800
2. Thomas Marketing Information Center (TMIC)
   One Penn Plaza
   Dept. TR
   New York, NY 10119
   (212) 290-7237
3. W. S. Ponton, Inc.
   The Ponton Building
   5149 Butler Street
   Pittsburgh, PA 15201
   1-800-628-7806

4. Ducker Research Co., Inc.
   6905-T Telegraph Road
   Birmingham, MI 48010
   (313) 644-0086

Good market consultants will identify who your competition is, how much of your product's market share each competitor currently holds, and how much market share you can hope to gain in specific incremental periods if you follow a particular marketing strategy. They can also identify best potential markets, pricing strategy, consumer acceptance of the product, and packaging. They can help determine which forms of advertising, and in what media, your particular product would be best promoted.

The services that a reputable marketing consultant can supply are almost endless. That is why it is extremely important for you to focus on just what kind of information you require to help get your product successfully on the shelf.

If you decide that hiring a marketing consultant is just too expensive or that you don't have sufficient background to work with the "raw" numbers available through one of the national marketing companies, and you find the hit-or-miss approach too chancy, there is one other option you might consider. Many small food companies are manufacturing their products successfully while operating their equipment at a very small percentage of production capability. They are often willing to contract out the manufacturing of a product. For example, Company A, which manufactures applesauce, is currently running a full shift (6 employees, 8 hours per day, 5 days per week). This production schedule allows the owner to fill all orders and keep an adequate inventory to supply his consistent growth pattern. Company B has a fruit-based ice cream topping product that requires the same processing and packaging equipment that Company A uses. An agreement is made for Company A to produce the topping for Company B in a large enough quantity to test the market without Company B having to commit enormous amounts of capital to a relatively risky venture. Keep in mind that less than 10% of the new food items launched each year are successful and, in 1987, there were over 10,000 new items tested! Your local chamber of commerce can be very helpful in identifying a local food processor with a complementary, but *not* competitive, food product who might be willing to contract the processing and/or packaging of your product.

What if, after you've done all your strategizing, the market won't take your product at the established price? If the market will not accept your product at a price which will cover your costs and the desired profit margin, you may do one of several things: discontinue manufacturing the product, accept a lower profit margin, reduce costs (labor, cost of raw materials, quality of packaging), or differentiate your product from your competitor's in the minds of the buyers. The first three choices are pretty basic. If you can lower your profit requirement, or if you can reduce costs enough to substantially lower your price, the market may accept your product. The fourth choice, product differentiation, is the one pricing option seldom used by small food manufacturers because it is so difficult to find that "unique" niche. If you can develop your product in such a way that perceived quality or perceived uniqueness of packaging make it a more marketable item, then you don't have to be as concerned with price. You can stress the nonprice factors in promoting and selling your product. A good example of this is the Pringles potato chip story. The processing costs for this particular product do not make it possible to compete in price with the more generic style potato chip brands, but the packaging is unique for potato chips. It offers the convenience of protecting the product during recreational outings or any event that requires additional transporting and handling of the product. It, therefore, fills a "unique" niche in the mind of the consumer.

CHAPTER 3

Organizing Your Business

Okay. So now you know what you want to produce and why. You even have a pretty good idea of how it's going to look when you're finished and how you're going to get it to your customer. Now, the process that is usually the least attractive to the entrepreneur must be handled . . . organizing your business.

This is the time when you need to take two steps back and do some heavy soul searching. The fun is over. Now it starts to get tough—but hey, if it was easy to start a business, everyone would do it.

Every year in the U.S. over half a million people, like yourself, decide to take the leap. The desire to be their own boss, make their own decisions, and control their own destiny gives them the incentive to launch their own business. Unfortunately, over one-half of these businesses will fail within the first 5 years of operation. Survival is especially tough in today's economy, with the small business beset on all sides by fluctuating money conditions, rising costs, uncertain supply sources, and erratic markets. If the right decisions are not made at this point, a new owner can lose everything—car, home, savings.

Without putting a real damper on your enthusiasm, you also need to be aware that owning a business (even a really profitable one) is not always as wonderful as it may seem. When you're the boss you may have many responsibilities that the people working for you don't have. The head of a business, particularly a relatively new business, often works 12 to 15 hours a day, 7 days a week. You shoulder the responsibility of employees, customers, suppliers, etc. You forfeit the right to a regular paycheck, a 40-hour work week, paid vacations, retirement security, and the attractive benefit packages offered by corporate America.

For a person with stamina, maturity, and creativity, for one who is willing to make sacrifices and take risks, an exhilarating and quite probably a financially rewarding experience awaits. Just make sure you give a lot of time and effort to this portion of your business strategy. Follow all the right steps and you are halfway there.

Planning Your Business

Figuring the amount of money it is going to take to set up your business is one of the most difficult parts of starting a business for many new entrepreneurs. It is absolutely essential that you figure *all* costs. Insufficient financing is a major cause of small business failure.

You must figure dollar requirements for the following:

- Purchase or lease of processing and packaging equipment
- Deposit on a lease or down payment on the purchase of a manufacturing facility
- Initial raw materials and packaging inventory
- Telephone and utility installation fees
- Stationary and office supply costs
- Taxes and licenses
- Advertising and promotional costs
- Insurance premiums
- Professional services (accountant, attorney, various consultants)

Along with these start-up costs, such operating expenses as owner and employee wages must be covered until the business shows a profit. Since many businesses take several months, if not years, to show a profit, at least enough funds should be available to cover the first 6 to 8 months of operation with additional cash built in for emergencies.

As you begin to move from the conceptual stage toward the actual formation of your new food processing operation, you need to answer the following questions:

- How much money is needed? Where will it come from?
- How much control do you want to have over operation? Are there portions of the operation (such as production, sales, accounting) that you would like to have control over, while leaving other portions under a more qualified person's control?
- What business skills might you lack that are needed for the entire operation?
- To what extent will you be personally responsible for debts or liabilities?
- How will the business be taxed?
- What will happen to the business if you are incapacitated for any length of time?

Your answers to these questions are crucial. This part of the organizational process can make you want to chuck the whole idea and go fishing, but it's important. This stage of your planning is the base upon which all your other efforts will be structured. If you start with a shaky base, you are going to spend the next few years of your business development in building supports, whereas, if you structure a firm foundation at the outset, your future operation should function smoothly.

Keep in mind that the organization of your operation is going to be continually reviewed. You will change certain aspects of the structure as profit and growth change. The food processor who starts out as a sole proprietor may, at some point, lack sufficient capital. This is not always a bad sign. Often extra dollars are needed to launch into a major new market. You may eventually seek a partner with available funds and complementary skills. Further down the road, if all goes well, you and your partner may decide to incorporate. All three forms of business ownership are open to you.

The following is an explanation, in very general terms, of some of the things you will need to know about starting your business. Please be aware, however, that no one expects you to do this alone. Be smart. Get help. There is all manner of expert, professional help available, often at little or no cost. Talk to your banker. Contact your local college or university to find out what kind of services they have to offer. Educate thyself! A list of state and federal organizations just waiting to help you appears at the end of this volume (see Appendices A, B, and C). So let's get started. This is your synopsis of Business 101.

Sole Proprietorship

When one person finances a business using only his or her cash (and possibly loans) the business is legally called a sole proprietorship. (Entrepreneurs love this one because they get to be totally in charge—but, they also get to have *all* the problems.) The sole proprietor makes or breaks the business which, as I mentioned, may sound singularly appealing to those instilled with the red-blooded American entrepreneurial spirit. It is difficult, however, to go it alone. The sole proprietor has sole control and sole responsibility. This person must provide or procure all the capital necessary to operate the business and is personally liable for all claims against the business.

On the positive side, the sole proprietorship is easy to initiate and is the least regulated form of business. The major advantage of the sole proprietorship is its simplicity. Organization costs and formalities are minimal. Unless a trade name is to be used (which, in most states, will require the filing of a trade name or doing-business certificate), or unless a special operating license is required by some government agency, few start-up or continuing formalities are necessary. The simplicity of the sole proprietorship means few technicalities in the continuing operation of the business. There are no shareholders, no board of directors, and no by-laws limiting your authority. Many of the tax and similar requirements to which corporations are normally subjected can be avoided. If you are planning on expanding and operating in other states you can do so without the formalities of corporation "qualifications," although you may have to file for a trade name or a doing-business certificate as requested by each individual state. Contact the state's small business agency to determine its requirements.

The major disadvantage of this form of business is the unlimited liability of the proprietor for all the debts of the business. In the event your business should fail, all of your non-business assets are subject to the claims of your creditors. Further, you can be held personally liable for tort claims (personal injuries or illness suffered by a consumer, for example). It is imperative that you protect yourself with a good insurance program (see Chapter 6).

Another disadvantage, from a family security vantage point, is that your business could collapse in the event of your illness or death. Bankers are sometimes uncomfortable with lending large sums to sole proprietors because of the possible disruption of business by death or disability of the owner. In addition, the lower rates that you will pay due to the nonapplicability of the usury laws to corporations make lending to sole proprietors less attractive.

Last, the poorer fringe benefits available to a sole proprietor must be considered. The tax advantages offered to corporations, particularly concerning pension and retirement plans, are not available to you. Sick pay, group insurance plans, death benefits, etc., are usually not available to you at an affordable rate. You should have a reliable banker or accountant explain the Keogh Retirement Plan to you as a form of retirement security for you and your family.

Sole proprietorship is appealing to someone who wants the business to stay small and simple. If you are considering keeping your production cost low by renting approved kitchen space and hand packaging, or by having your original inventory processed by an established manufacturer, you might want to try sole proprietorship. Setting up a food processing operation costs many dollars. Unless you are a millionaire or you are willing to take out major personal loans and deal with some of the other disadvantages mentioned, you will probably need to look at other options.

General Partnership

A general partnership is the pooling of resources and capital of two or more people, as co-owners, to conduct business. An "idea" person and a "money" person often provide the formula for a successful partnership. The general partnership is easy to set up, for it requires no official registration beyond that of any pseudonym the partners plan to use. Although a written agreement among partners is not required by law, it is wise to have an attorney draw up a contract which spells out the respective rights and duties of the partners. It is very important, even (or particularly) if you and your partner are "friends," to draw up a very detailed agreement as to who is in charge of what portions of the business and what your business goals are. As many partnerships quickly sour, you are better off finding a partner you respect and can work with on a neutral ground. You'll need your "friends" in the future!

Partnerships do not have to be fifty-fifty. Almost any management and profit-sharing arrangement is possible. The death or withdrawal of one partner or the addition of a new partner legally terminates a partnership. This may not necessarily mean liquidation of the business. A new contract can be drawn up, but be sure you make the necessary provisions for such a dissolution in the original written agreement. Make sure you have a good attorney—someone who has a background in working with entrepreneurs, someone you can trust. Taking care of these issues now ensures smooth transition of ownership and continuity of business operations.

A partnership is not a separate legal entity. Partnership liability extends to the personal assets of the general partners, and each partner is taxed on his or her share of the partnership income based on personal income tax rates.

This form of business has great potential for the entrepreneur food processor, particularly if he or she can find a partner who has a background in the food industry. The ideal situation would be to find a retired or soon-to-be-retired executive from a major food corporation who isn't quite ready to get out of the business. Kraft Foods (for example) has thousands of managers and Kroger Foods has a large number of grocery experts who might be interested in investing their time, knowledge, *contacts*, and money in a new food processing venture.

Limited Partnership

The limited partnership is often regarded as the *ideal* arrangement for the entrepreneur food processor. The limited partnership is a refinement of the principle of partnership. More closely regulated than the general partnership, it permits investors to become partners without assuming unlimited liability. There must be at least one general partner—you. The limited partner usually risks only as much as his or her original investment.

Corporation

According to Chief Justice John Marshall, "A corporation is an artificial being, invisible, intangible, and existing only in contemplation of the law." Now you ask yourself, "Say what?" Simply put, the corporation is set up to function as a separate entity—apart from the owners or shareholders. It makes contracts, it is liable, it pays taxes. It is a legal "entity." Even more simply, a corporation is set up to bear a lot of the burden, especially if your business falls short of your plans.

A corporation can attract capital by selling stock in the company to selected investors or to the public. However, you shouldn't be thinking about "going public" until you have established your business and have a track record to sell. This form of business should be considered when your operation is starting to require large amounts of capital, and you should get some expert guidance.

It can't be stressed enough how important it is to find a qualified tax consultant to help you make the right choices, particularly at this stage of your business development. A smart counselor will probably advise you to consider setting your business up under a Subchapter S Corporation.

Very simply put, a Subchapter S Corporation is a business corporation which elects to be treated like a partnership for tax reasons. It has all corporate powers except it is limited to 35 shareholders (restricted to U.S. citizens); the entity files IRS Form 1120S, allowing taxation of shareholders as individuals. The long and short of it is that you enjoy the limited liability of a corporation, but you avoid double taxation and are taxed like a partnership.

The key to using an S Corporation is foresight (and the support of a good tax advisor). You must anticipate your tax situation for the coming year. You cannot elect to be an S Corporation *after* realizing you need to be one.

Not all companies are eligible to be S Corporations. To be eligible, the corporation

1. Must not have more than 35 shareholders;
2. Must not have a corporation, a nonresident alien, a foreign trust, or certain other types of trusts as one of its shareholders; and,
3. Must not show more than 25% of its gross receipt as passive income (interest, royalties, rents).

If the company is eligible, it must file Form 2533 with the IRS by March 15 (all S Corporations must operate on the calendar year). On Form 2533, stockholders give their consent for the company to be taxed as a partnership.

There are a lot of technical details involving capital gains treatment, etc., and that is why you *must* have a good tax counselor if you decide to go this route. You must pay attention to *all* the details.

Taxes

After you decide how you are going to set up your business, you need to decide how you are going to handle the tax structure. The following is a brief overview of the various business taxes, but it can not be stressed firmly enough that, for this portion of your business development, you must get professional assitance. A good accountant, though expensive, will save you a lot of money and hassle in the long run. Contact your state's professional accountant association to get some names. Find one who has experience working with small food processors.

Keep in mind that the tax liability of a business is affected not only by the legal form of the business but by the myriad of other management decisions as well. That is one reason why a good accountant or attorney can be invaluable in helping you sort out your options. The following sections describe several types of taxes you will probably be responsible for.

Federal Income Taxes

For the sole proprietor, filing federal income tax returns is pretty basic. You simply list all business income and deductions in an individual income tax return (Form 1040) and file specific tax schedules relating to the business. Don't hesitate to contact your local IRS office for assistance (see Appendix C).

A partnership's income is taxed as personal income to the partners and each partner's distributive share is reported on his or her individual tax return. Save yourself a lot of hassle and have a good accountant handle this. The partnership's income must be filed for information purposes under federal law. Form 1065 is used for this federal information return.

Income and deductions of a corporation are computed at the corporate level, and taxes are paid on the corporation's taxable income. Most corporations file income tax returns on Form 1120. You may also be required to file an estimated tax payment (Form 1120W). Unless you have a strong accounting background, get yourself a good accountant!

State Income Taxes

Each state has different tax requirements for business. Contact your local state tax office.

Employment Taxes

The federal government generally requires every business with one or more employees to withhold federal income and social security taxes from all wages paid, including those paid to yourself. Don't try to avoid these taxes. If, and when, the government catches up with you, the penalties can be devastating.

The first thing you need to do is get an employer's identification number. This is required on all employment tax returns. All you have to do is fill out Form SS-4 (see Figure 3.1) with your local IRS center. This identification number is similar to, but not the same as, your Social Security number. When you file your form, request a copy of Circular E, Employer's Tax Guide (IRS Publication 15), which contains some excellent information on taxes. Much of this information is gleaned from the booklet.

State employment taxes vary from state to state. Again, contact your local office for information necessary in filing state employment tax.

Property Tax

Generally, all businesses must pay personal property tax once a year. You will have to pay personal property tax on

Form **SS-4** (Rev. August 1989) Department of the Treasury Internal Revenue Service	**Application for Employer Identification Number** (For use by employers and others. Please read the attached instructions before completing this form.) Please type or print clearly.	EIN OMB No. 1545-0003 Expires 7-31-91

1 Name of applicant (True legal name) (See instructions.)

2 Trade name of business, if different from name in line 1 | **3** Executor, trustee, "care of name"

4a Mailing address (street address) (room, apt., or suite no.) | **5a** Address of business. (See instructions.)

4b City, state, and ZIP code | **5b** City, state, and ZIP code

6 County and state where principal business is located

7 Name of principal officer, grantor, or general partner. (See instructions.) ▶

8a Type of entity (Check only one box.) (See instructions.)
☐ Individual SSN _____
☐ REMIC   ☐ Personal service corp.
☐ State/local government   ☐ National guard
☐ Other nonprofit organization (specify)_____
☐ Other (specify) ▶
☐ Estate
☐ Plan administrator SSN _____
☐ Other corporation (specify) _____
☐ Federal government/military
If nonprofit organization enter GEN (if applicable)_____
☐ Trust
☐ Partnership
☐ Farmers' cooperative
☐ Church or church controlled organization

8b If a corporation, give name of foreign country (if applicable) or state in the U.S. where incorporated ▶ | Foreign country | State

9 Reason for applying (Check only one box)
☐ Started new business
☐ Hired employees
☐ Created a pension plan (specify type) ▶
☐ Banking purpose (specify) ▶
☐ Changed type of organization (specify) ▶_____
☐ Purchased going business
☐ Created a trust (specify) ▶_____
☐ Other (specify) ▶

10 Date business started or acquired (Mo., day, year) (See instructions.) | **11** Enter closing month of accounting year. (See instructions.)

12 First date wages or annuities were paid or will be paid (Mo., day, year). **Note:** If applicant is a withholding agent, enter date income will first be paid to nonresident alien. (Mo., day, year). ▶

13 Enter highest number of employees expected in the next 12 months. **Note:** If the applicant does not expect to have any employees during the period, enter "0". ▶ | Nonagricultural | Agricultural | Household

14 Does the applicant operate more than one place of business? . . . . ☐ Yes ☐ No
If "Yes," enter name of business. ▶

15 Principal activity or service (See instructions.) ▶

16 Is the principal business activity manufacturing? . . . . ☐ Yes ☐ No
If "Yes," principal product and raw material used ▶

17 To whom are most of the products or services sold? Please check the appropriate box.   ☐ Business (wholesale)
☐ Public (retail)   ☐ Other (specify) ▶   ☐ N/A

18a Has the applicant ever applied for an identification number for this or any other business? . . . . ☐ Yes ☐ No
Note: If "Yes," please complete lines 18b and 18c.

18b If you checked the "Yes" box in line 18a, give applicant's true name and trade name, if different than name shown on prior application.

True name ▶   Trade name ▶

18c Enter approximate date, city, and state where the application was filed and the previous employer identification number if known.

Approximate date when filed (Mo., day, year) | City and state where filed | Previous EIN

Under penalties of perjury, I declare that I have examined this application, and to the best of my knowledge and belief, it is true, correct, and complete. | Telephone number (include area code)

Name and title (Please type or print clearly.) ▶

Signature ▶   Date ▶

Note: Do not write below this line.   For official use only.

Please leave blank ▶	Geo.	Ind.	Class	Size	Reason for applying

For Paperwork Reduction Act Notice, see attached instructions.   ☆U.S. Government Printing Office: 1989-262-151/80163   Form **SS-4** (Rev. 8-89)

Figure 3.1   SS-4. Application for employer identification number.

equipment, supplies, office furnishings, and the like. You will also be responsible for real property tax on your land and building if you own your processing facility.

Some of the tax credits you might need to know about are described in the following sections.

Investment Tax Credit

The investment tax credit is one of the federal income tax provisions important to new businesses. This provision allows you to take a tax credit on up to 10% of the first $125,000 invested in used property. The credit applies only to certain property and the property must have a useful life of at least 3 years to be eligible for any portion of the credit. Many states have their own tax credits for new businesses. Talk to your accountant!

Rehabilitation Expenditures Credit

Expenditures on the rehabilitation of buildings in use for a specified period that have not been rehabilitated during that period may qualify for a tax credit. Again, talk to your accountant.

Business Energy Investment Credit

Businesses are allowed to claim a tax credit of from 10 to 15% on qualified investments in energy property. This can be helpful if you are involved in aquaculture, greenhouse production, or dehydration through solar use.

Table 3.1 is a very helpful tax matrix which was developed by Coopers and Lybrand, an outstanding accounting company.

Tax Forms

Completing this section on taxes are examples of some of the tax forms you may need and a brief summary of each.

W-4 Employee's Withholding Allowance Certificate

The W-4 Form (Figure 3.2) allows your employee to fix the amount of tax withheld from his wages to his tax liability by claiming an appropriate number of deductions, so that the employer may withhold the proper amount of tax in each pay period. Any person you employ in your food processing operation may be required to file an annual income tax return and regardless of whether they are required to file you <u>must</u> have this completed form on file.

W-2 Wage and Tax Statement

The W-2 Form (Figure 3.3a) and W-2P (Figure 3.3b) are official records of the amount of wages or other compensation you have paid your employee. It shows the amount of federal and state income tax withheld as well as FICA tax withheld. You must give all employees a completed W-2 by January 31 of each year for their income tax returns. (See Figure 3.3c for instructions.)

1099 Miscellaneous Statement for Recipients of Non-Employee Compensation

This is the form you will need to complete if you are your only employee (Figure 3.4). It is a formal record of annual earnings for the self-employed.

941 Employer's Quarterly Federal Tax Return

This form is used to report income tax withheld from wages, annuities, supplemental unemployment compensation benefits, and taxes under the federal insurance contribution (Figure 3.5). If you withhold income tax and FICA from your employees' wages, you must file this return on the last day of the month following the close of the reporting quarter.

Table 3.1[a]
Comparisons of Various Forms of Doing Business

TREATMENT OF INCOME AND EXPENSES	Proprietorship	Partnership	Regular Corporation	S Corporation
Character of Income and deductions	Tax attributes are reflected in the individual's return, and maintain their identity.	Conduit—no tax to partnership.	Taxed at corporate level.	Conduit—could be passive income. Potential corporate built-in or capital gains taxes.
Capital gain	Capital gains will be taxed as ordinary capital gains.	Conduit—taxed as capital gains at the partner level.	Taxed as ordinary income.	Possible corporate capital gains or built-in gains tax; conduit—taxed as capital gains at the shareholder level.
Capital loss	Limited to $3,000 per year; excess is carried forward indefinitely. Losses offset ordinary income on a dollar-for-dollar basis.	Conduit—limitation apply at the partner level.	Carry back three years and carry over five years as short-term capital loss offsetting only capital gains.	Conduit—limitations apply at the shareholder level.
Section 1231 gains and losses	Taxed at individual level, combined with other Section 1231 gains or losses of individual; net gains are capital; net losses are ordinary.	Conduit—limitations apply at the partner level; taxed as ordinary income.	Taxable or deductible at the corporate level.	Possible corporate capital gains or built-in gains tax; conduit—limitations apply at the shareholder level; taxed as ordinary income.
Expensing of depreciable business assets	Election to expense is allowed up to $10,000 a year. Expensing allowance phases out dollar for dollar when the cost of qualified property placed in service during the taxable year is between $200,000-$210,000.	Same.	Same.	Same.
Organization costs	Not amortizable.	Amortizable over 60 months.	Amortizable over 60 months.	Amortizable over 60 months.
Charitable contributions	Subject to limits for individual: Generally, gifts to public charity, cash 50% of AGI; appreciated property 30% of AGI. Other limitations for specific items contributed. Unused portion may be carried forward five years.	Conduit—limitations apply at the partner level.	Deduction is limited to 10% of modified taxable income. Unused portion may be carried forward five years.	Conduit—limitations apply at the shareholder level.
Dividends received	Treated as ordinary income, no exclusion or deduction. Portfolio taint retained.	Conduit with portfolio taint retained.	80% to 100% dividend-received deduction. Special rules on portfolio income for closely-held corporations.	Conduit with portfolio taint retained.
Alternative minimum tax	For individuals, the alternative minimum tax rate is 24%. The exemption amount is determined by filing status and alternative minimum taxable income.	Conduit for preference items. The alternative minimum tax is calculated at the partner level.	For corporate taxpayers, the alternative minimum tax rate is 20%. The alternative minimum tax is imposed on alternative minimum taxable income in excess of $40,000, but only if the amount is more than the regular corporate tax. ATM may be applied as a credit against future regular tax.	Conduit for preference items. The alternative minimum tax is calculated at the shareholder level.

Table 3.1 (continues)

[a]Reprinted with permission of Coopers and Lybrand

	Proprietorship	Partnership	Regular Corporation	S Corporation
TREATMENT OF INCOME AND EXPENSES				
Tax preferences	Depletion, accelerated depreciation, excess drilling costs, passive losses, net unrealized gain on certain charitable contributions, among others.	Conduct—preference items separately stated and reflected in the calculation of AMT at the partner level. No book-tax preference.	Adjusted current earnings (ACE) adjustment, depletion, accelerated depreciation, net unrealized gain on certain charitable contributions, among others.	Conduct—preference items separately stated and reflected in the calculation of AMT at the partner level. No ACE adjustment.
Accounting methods	Cash or accrual.	Cash or accrual, but partnership with C corporation partners with more then $5 million gross receipts and tax shelter partnerships cannot use cash method.	Accrual, but cash available to C corporations with $5 million or less gross receipts.	Cash or accrual.
TREATMENT OF COMPENSATION AND BENEFITS				
Partner's or shareholders "reasonable" salary	Not applicable.	Can be deductible by partnership or treated as an allocation of partnership profits.	Deductible by the corporation and taxable to the shareholder-employee.	Deductible by the corporation and taxable to the shareholder-employee.
Group hospitalization and life insurance premiums and medical reimbursement plans	Medical expenses are an itemized deduction. Only medical expenses exceeding 7.5% of adjusted gross income will be deductible. Self-employed individuals can deduct up to 25% of their medical insurance premiums through 1991 unless they are covered by a qualified plan. No deduction is allowed for life insurance premiums.	Cost of partner's benefits generally not deductible by partnership. May be treated as a distribution to individual partners, eligible for possible deduction at partner level. Partners can deduct up to 25% of their medical insurance premiums through 1991, unless they are covered by a qualified plan.	Cost of shareholder-employee's coverage is generally deductible as a business expense if the plan is a qualified plan "for the benefit of employees."	Same as partnership for more than 2% shareholders, including eligibility to deduct up to 25% of their medical insurance premiums through 1991.
Retirement benefits	Limitations and restrictions basically same as regular corporation.	Limitations and restrictions basically same as regular corporation.	Limitations on benefits from defined benefit plans - lesser $90,000 (adjusted for cost of living increases) or 100% of compensation.	Limitation on contributions basically the same as a regular corporation.
ALLOCATIONS, DISTRIBUTIONS AND LOSS LIMITATIONS				
Basis of allocating operating income or loss to owners	All income or loss picked up on owner's return.	Partnership profit and loss agreement (may have "special allocations" of income and deductions if they reflect economic reality).	No income allocated to stockholders.	Pro-rata portion of income or loss and separately stated items, based on per share, per day allocation.
Distributions to owners	Drawings from the business are not taxable; the net profits are taxable; and the proprietor is subject to the tax on self-employment income.	Generally not taxable.	Payment of salaries are deductible by corporation and taxable to recipient; payments of dividends are not deductible by corporation and generally are taxable to recipient shareholders.	Payments of salaries deductible by corporation and taxable to recipient; distributions generally not taxable.
Limitations on losses deductible by owners • basis • at-risk • passive loss	• Not applicable • Limited to amount at-risk • Passive loss limitations apply to owner.	• Limited to Partner's basis (including entity level debt) • Limited to amount at-risk • Passive loss limitation apply at the partner level.	• No losses allowed to individual, except upon sale of stock or liquidation of the corporation. • Certain closely-held corporations subject to passive loss limitations.	• Limited to shareholder's basis (contributions to capital plus loans to corporation). • Limited to amount "at risk." • Passive loss limitations apply at the shareholder level.

Table 3.1 (continues)

STRUCTURE OF OWNERSHIP	Proprietorship	Partnership	Regular Corporation	S Corporation
Formal election required	No.	No, but a partnership agreement should be drafted.	Must incorporate under state law.	Yes.
Qualified owners	Individual ownership.	No limitation.	No limitation.	Individual citizens, resident aliens, estates and certain trusts may be shareholders. Number of shareholders limited to 35.
Type of ownership interest	Individual ownership.	More than one class of partner permitted.	More than one class of stock permitted.	Only one class of stock permitted.
Transfer of ownership	Assets of business transferable rather than business itself.	Consent of other partners often required if partnership interest is to be transferred, depending upon partnership agreement. New partnership may be created.	Ready transfer of ownership through the use of stock certificates; restrictions may be imposed by shareholder's agreement.	Shares can be transferred only to certain individuals, certain types of trusts, or estates. No consent is needed by a new shareholder for S election.
Taxable year	Usually calendar year.	Must have a calendar year unless there is a business purpose, i.e., a natural business year.	Any year is permissible upon adoption, changes require business purposes. Special rules apply to personal service corporations.	Must have a calendar year unless there is a business purpose, i.e., a natural business year.
Flexibility	No restrictions.	Partnership is contractual arrangement, within which members can do in business what individuals can, subject to the partnership agreement and applicable state laws.	Corporation is a creature of the state functioning with powers granted explicitly or necessarily implied, subject to judicial construction and decisions.	Same as regular corporation.
Capital requirements	Capital raised only by loan or increased contribution by proprietor.	Loans or contributions from partners (original, or newly created by remaking partnership).	Met by sale of stock, issuance of bonds, or by taking on other corporate debt.	Met by sale of stock or issuance of debt, but corporation can issue only one class of stock and is limited to 35 shareholders.
GENERAL	Proprietorship	Partnership	Regular Corporation	S Corporation
Liability	Individual is liable on all liabilities of the business.	General partners individually liable on partnership liabilities. Limited partners liable only up to amount of his or her unpaid capital contributions, plus distributions in the last year (in many states).	Shareholder's liability limited to capital contributions.	Same as regular.
Business action	Sole proprietor makes decisions and can act immediately.	Action dependent upon the agreement of partners or general partners, as defined in the partnership agreement.	Unity of action based on authority or board of directors.	Same as regular corporation, except unanimous consent is required to elect S corporation status. more than 50% of shareholders needed to revoke S status, however, can be revoked by failure to meet requirements.
Management	Proprietor is responsible and recognizes all profits or losses.	Except for limited or silent partners, investment in partnership involves responsibility for management decisions.	Shareholder can receive dividends without sharing in responsibility for management.	Shareholders entitled to allocable shares of income and income items without responsibility for management decisions.

Table 3.1 (continued)

1991 Form W-4

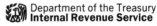
Department of the Treasury
Internal Revenue Service

Purpose. Complete Form W-4 so that your employer can withhold the correct amount of Federal income tax from your pay.
Exemption From Withholding. Read line 6 of the certificate below to see if you can claim exempt status. *If exempt, complete line 6; but do not complete lines 4 and 5.* No Federal income tax will be withheld from your pay. Your exemption is good for one year only. It expires February 15, 1992.
Basic Instructions. Employees who are not exempt should complete the Personal Allowances Worksheet. Additional worksheets are provided on page 2 for employees to adjust their withholding allowances based on itemized deductions, adjustments to income, or two-earner/two-job situations. Complete all worksheets that apply to your situation. The worksheets will help you figure the number of withholding allowances you are

entitled to claim. However, you may claim fewer allowances than this.
Head of Household. Generally, you may claim head of household filing status on your tax return only if you are unmarried and pay more than 50% of the costs of keeping up a home for yourself and your dependent(s) or other qualifying individuals.
Nonwage Income. If you have a large amount of nonwage income, such as interest or dividends, you should consider making estimated tax payments using Form 1040-ES. Otherwise, you may find that you owe additional tax at the end of the year.
Two-Earner/Two-Jobs. If you have a working spouse or more than one job, figure the total number of allowances you are entitled to claim on all jobs using worksheets from only one Form

W-4. This total should be divided among all jobs. Your withholding will usually be most accurate when all allowances are claimed on the W-4 filed for the highest paying job and zero allowances are claimed for the others.
Advance Earned Income Credit. If you are eligible for this credit, you can receive it added to your paycheck throughout the year. For details, get Form W-5 from your employer.
Check Your Withholding. After your W-4 takes effect, you can use **Pub. 919,** Is My Withholding Correct for 1991?, to see how the dollar amount you are having withheld compares to your estimated total annual tax. Call 1-800-829-3676 to order this publication. Check your local telephone directory for the IRS assistance number if you need further help.

Personal Allowances Worksheet For 1991, the value of your personal exemption(s) is reduced if your income is over $100,000 ($150,000 if married filing jointly, $125,000 if head of household, or $75,000 if married filing separately). Get Pub. 919 for details.

A Enter "1" for **yourself** if no one else can claim you as a dependent . . . . **A** ____

B Enter "1" if: { **1.** You are single and have only one job; or
2. You are married, have only one job, and your spouse does not work; or
3. Your wages from a second job or your spouse's wages (or the total of both) are $1,000 or less. } **B** ____

C Enter "1" for your **spouse.** But, you may choose to enter "0" if you are married and have either a working spouse or more than one job (this may help you avoid having too little tax withheld) . . . . **C** ____

D Enter number of **dependents** (other than your spouse or yourself) whom you will claim on your tax return . . . . . **D** ____

E Enter "1" if you will file as **head of household** on your tax return (see conditions under "Head of Household," above) . . **E** ____

F Enter "1" if you have at least $1,500 of **child or dependent care expenses** for which you plan to claim a credit . . . **F** ____

G Add lines A through F and enter total here . . . . ▶ **G** ____

For accuracy, do all worksheets that apply.
• If you plan to **itemize or claim adjustments to income** and want to reduce your withholding, see the Deductions and Adjustments Worksheet on page 2.
• If you are **single** and have **more than one job** and your combined earnings from all jobs exceed $27,000 OR if you are **married** and have a **working spouse or more than one job**, and the combined earnings from all jobs exceed $46,000, see the Two-Earner/Two-Job Worksheet on page 2 if you want to avoid having too little tax withheld.
• If **neither** of the above situations applies, **stop here** and enter the number from line G on line 4 of Form W-4 below.

-------------------- Cut here and give the certificate to your employer. Keep the top portion for your records. --------------------

Form **W-4**
Department of the Treasury
Internal Revenue Service

Employee's Withholding Allowance Certificate
▶ **For Privacy Act and Paperwork Reduction Act Notice, see reverse.**

OMB No. 1545-0010

1991

1 Type or print your first name and middle initial	Last name	2 Your social security number

Home address (number and street or rural route)	3 Marital status	☐ Single ☐ Married ☐ Married, but withhold at higher Single rate.
City or town, state, and ZIP code		**Note:** *If married, but legally separated, or spouse is a nonresident alien, check the Single box.*

4 Total number of allowances you are claiming (from line G above or from the Worksheets on back if they apply) . . . . **4** ____

5 Additional amount, if any, you want deducted from each pay . . . . **5** $ ____

6 I claim exemption from withholding and I certify that I meet **ALL** of the following conditions for exemption:
 • Last year I had a right to a refund of **ALL** Federal income tax withheld because I had **NO** tax liability; **AND**
 • This year I expect a refund of **ALL** Federal income tax withheld because I expect to have **NO** tax liability; **AND**
 • This year if my income exceeds $550 and includes nonwage income, another person cannot claim me as a dependent.
If you meet all of the above conditions, enter the year effective and "EXEMPT" here . . . . . ▶ **6** 19__

7 Are you a full-time student? (**Note:** *Full-time students are not automatically exempt.*) . . . . **7** ☐ Yes ☐ No

Under penalties of perjury, I certify that I am entitled to the number of withholding allowances claimed on this certificate or entitled to claim exempt status.

Employee's signature ▶ _____ Date ▶ _____ , 19__

8 Employer's name and address (**Employer: Complete 8 and 10 only if sending to IRS**)	9 Office code (optional)	10 Employer identification number

Figure 3.2 W-4 form. Employee's withholding allowance certificate.

Taxes

Deductions and Adjustments Worksheet

Note: *Use this worksheet only if you plan to itemize deductions or claim adjustments to income on your 1991 tax return.*

1 Enter an estimate of your 1991 itemized deductions. These include: qualifying home mortgage interest, charitable contributions, state and local taxes (but not sales taxes), medical expenses in excess of 7.5% of your income, and miscellaneous deductions. (For 1991, you may have to reduce your itemized deductions if your income is over $100,000 ($50,000 if married filing separately). Get Pub. 919 for details.) . . . . . **1** $ _____

2 Enter: { $5,700 if married filing jointly or qualifying widow(er) / $5,000 if head of household / $3,400 if single / $2,850 if married filing separately } . . . . **2** $ _____

3 **Subtract** line 2 from line 1. If line 2 is greater than line 1, enter zero. . . . . **3** $ _____

4 Enter an estimate of your 1991 adjustments to income. These include alimony paid and deductible IRA contributions . . **4** $ _____

5 **Add** lines 3 and 4 and enter the total . . . . **5** $ _____

6 Enter an estimate of your 1991 nonwage income (such as dividends or interest income) . . . . . **6** $ _____

7 **Subtract** line 6 from line 5. Enter the result, but not less than zero . . . . **7** $ _____

8 **Divide** the amount on line 7 by $2,000 and enter the result here. Drop any fraction. . . . . . **8** _____

9 Enter the number from Personal Allowances Worksheet, line G, on page 1 . . . . **9** _____

10 **Add** lines 8 and 9 and enter the total here. If you use the Two-Earner/Two-Job Worksheet, also enter the total on line 1, below. Otherwise, **stop here** and enter this total on Form W-4, line 4 on page 1 . . . **10** _____

Two-Earner/Two-Job Worksheet

Note: *Use this worksheet only if the instructions for line G on page 1 direct you here.*

1 Enter the number from line G on page 1 (or from line 10 above if you used the Deductions and Adjustments Worksheet) . **1** _____

2 Find the number in **Table 1** below that applies to the **LOWEST** paying job and enter it here . . . . . **2** _____

3 If line 1 is **GREATER THAN OR EQUAL TO** line 2, subtract line 2 from line 1. Enter the result here (if zero, enter "0") and on Form W-4, line 4, on page 1. **DO NOT** use the rest of this worksheet . . . . **3** _____

Note: *If line 1 is **LESS THAN** line 2, enter "0" on Form W-4, line 4, on page 1. Complete lines 4–9 to calculate the additional dollar withholding necessary to avoid a year-end tax bill.*

4 Enter the number from line 2 of this worksheet . . . . **4** _____

5 Enter the number from line 1 of this worksheet . . . . **5** _____

6 **Subtract** line 5 from line 4 . . . . **6** _____

7 Find the number in **Table 2** below that applies to the **HIGHEST** paying job and enter it here . . . . **7** $ _____

8 **Multiply** line 7 by line 6 and enter the result here. This is the additional annual withholding amount needed **8** $ _____

9 Divide line 8 by the number of pay periods remaining in 1991. (For example, divide by 26 if you are paid every other week and you complete this form in December of 1990.) Enter the result here and on Form W-4, line 5, page 1. This is the additional amount to be withheld from each paycheck . . . . **9** $ _____

Table 1: Two-Earner/Two-Job Worksheet

Married Filing Jointly		All Others	
If wages from **LOWEST** paying job are—	Enter on line 2 above	If wages from **LOWEST** paying job are—	Enter on line 2 above
0 - $4,000	0	0 - $6,000	0
4,001 - 8,000	1	6,001 - 10,000	1
8,001 - 12,000	2	10,001 - 14,000	2
12,001 - 17,000	3	14,001 - 18,000	3
17,001 - 21,000	4	18,001 - 22,000	4
21,001 - 26,000	5	22,001 - 45,000	5
26,001 - 30,000	6	45,001 and over	6
30,001 - 35,000	7		
35,001 - 40,000	8		
40,001 - 55,000	9		
55,001 - 75,000	10		
75,001 and over	11		

Table 2: Two-Earner/Two-Job Worksheet

Married Filing Jointly		All Others	
If wages from **HIGHEST** paying job are—	Enter on line 7 above	If wages from **HIGHEST** paying job are—	Enter on line 7 above
0 - $46,000	$320	0 - $26,000	$320
46,001 - 94,000	600	26,001 - 55,000	600
94,001 and over	670	55,001 and over	670

Privacy Act and Paperwork Reduction Act Notice.—We ask for the information on this form to carry out the Internal Revenue laws of the United States. The Internal Revenue Code requires this information under sections 3402(f)(2)(A) and 6109 and their regulations. Failure to provide a completed form will result in your being treated as a single person who claims no withholding allowances. Routine uses of this information include giving it to the Department of Justice for civil and criminal litigation and to cities, states, and the District of Columbia for use in administering their tax laws.

The time needed to complete this form will vary depending on individual circumstances. The estimated average time is: **Recordkeeping** 46 min., **Learning about the law or the form** 10 min., **Preparing the form** 70 min. If you have comments concerning the accuracy of these time estimates or suggestions for making this form more simple, we would be happy to hear from you. You can write to both the **Internal Revenue Service**, Washington, DC 20224, Attention: IRS Reports Clearance Officer, T:FP; and the **Office of Management and Budget**, Paperwork Reduction Project (1545-0010), Washington, DC 20503. **DO NOT** send the tax form to either of these offices. Instead, give it to your employer.

☆U.S. GOVERNMENT PRINTING OFFICE: 1990-265-086

Figure 3.2 *(continued).*

(a)

1 Control number		OMB No 1545-0008						
2 Employer's name, address, and ZIP code			6 Statutory employee ☐	Deceased ☐	Pension plan ☐	Legal rep ☐	942 emp ☐	Subtotal ☐	Deferred compensation ☐	Void ☐
			7 Allocated tips			8 Advance EIC payment		
3 Employer's identification number	4 Employer's state I.D. number		9 Federal income tax withheld			10 Wages, tips, other compensation		
5 Employee's social security number			11 Social security tax withheld			12 Social security wages		
19a Employee's name (first, middle, last)			13 Social security tips			14 Nonqualified plans		
			15 Dependent care benefits			16 Fringe benefits incl. in Box 10		
			17			18 Other		
19b Employee's address and ZIP code								
20	21		22			23		
24 State income tax	25 State wages, tips. etc.	26 Name of state	27 Local income tax		28 Local wages, tips. etc.	29 Name of locality		

Copy B To be filed with employee's FEDERAL tax return

Form W-2 Wage and Tax Statement 1990

Dept. of the Treasury—Internal Revenue Service

This information is being furnished to the Internal Revenue Service

Figure 3.3a *W-2 form. Wage and tax statement.*

52

(b)

1 Control number		For Official Use Only ▶ OMB No. 1545-0008		
55555				

2 Payer's name, address, and ZIP code	3 Payer's Federal identification number	4 Payer's state I.D. number
	5 State income tax withheld	6 Name of state

7 Tax amt not determined ☐	Deceased ☐	Legal rep. ☐	Subtotal ☐	IRA/SEP ☐	Void ☐

8 Recipient's social security no.	9 Gross annuity, pension, etc.	10 Taxable amount	11 Federal income tax withheld

12 Recipient's name (first, middle, last)	13	14 Distribution code

For Paperwork Reduction Act Notice, see separate instructions.

Copy A—For Social Security Administration
See Instructions for Forms W-2 and W-2P and back of Copy D.

15 Recipient's address and ZIP code

Form **W-2P** **1990**   **Statement for Recipients of Annuities, Pensions, Retired Pay, or IRA Payments**   Department of the Treasury Internal Revenue Service

Do NOT Cut or Separate Forms on This Page

Figure 3.3b   W-2P. Statement for recipients of annuities, pensions, retired pay, or IRA payments.

(c)

Instructions

Please use this form to report payments under a retirement plan. Examples are pensions, retainer pay, annuities under a purchased contract, and payments from individual retirement accounts or annuities. See the separate **Instructions for Forms W-2 and W-2P** for more information on how to complete Form W-2P.

Use Form W-2 to report payments that are subject to social security tax.

You need not file Form W-2P for the following cases: (a) You paid retirement benefits that are exempt from tax such as Department of Veterans Affairs payments; (b) You made payments as a fiduciary, filed Form 1041, and gave each beneficiary a Schedule K-1 (Form 1041); (c) You made total distributions reported on Form 1099-R.

Figure 3.3c   Instructions for W-2 and W-2P forms.

9595	☐ VOID	☐ CORRECTED				
Type or machine print PAYER'S name, street address, city, state, and ZIP code			1 Rents $	OMB No. 1545-0115		Miscellaneous Income
			2 Royalties $	1990		
			3 Prizes, awards, etc. $	Statement for Recipients of		
PAYER'S Federal identification number	RECIPIENT'S identification number		4 Federal income tax withheld $	5 Fishing boat proceeds $		Copy A For Internal
Type or machine print RECIPIENT'S name			6 Medical and health care payments $	7 Nonemployee compensation $		Revenue Service Center
Street address			8 Substitute payments in lieu of dividends or interest $	9 Payer made direct sales of $5,000 or more of consumer products to a buyer (recipient) for resale ▶ ☐		For Paperwork Reduction Act Notice and instructions for completing this
City, state, and ZIP code			10 Crop insurance proceeds $	11 State income tax withheld $		form, see Instructions for Forms 1099,
Account number (optional)			12 State/Payer's state number			1098, 5498, and W-2G.

Form 1099-MISC

Do NOT Cut or Separate Forms on This Page

Department of the Treasury - Internal Revenue Service

Figure 3.4   1099-Miscellaneous form.

940 Employer's Annual Federal Unemployment Tax Return

This form, (Figure 3.6) is used for annual reporting of tax under the Federal Unemployment Act. The tax is paid only by you, the employer. If you pay wages of at least $1500 in any calendar quarter or at any time had one or more employees in any 20 calendar weeks, you have to file this return.

W-3 Transmittal of Income and Tax Statements

Your government at its best! This form (Figure 3.7) must accompany, and organizes, filings of Forms W-2 and W-2P into categories, as shown on the form. If you have to file W-2 or W-2P, you have to file W-3.

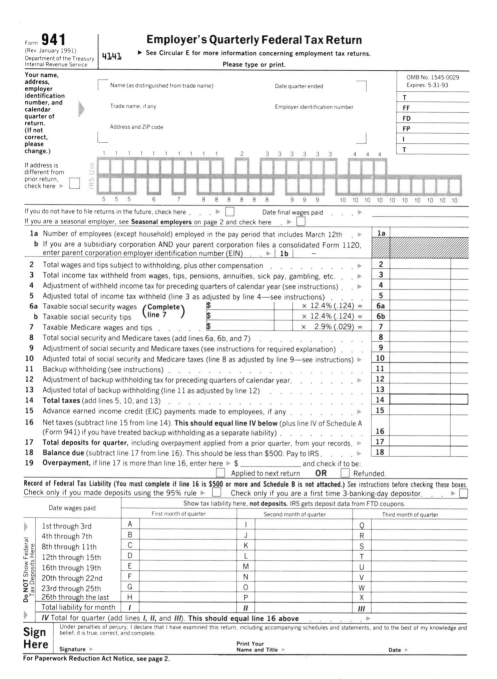

Figure 3.5 941 form. Employer's quarterly federal tax return.

Form **940**

Department of the Treasury
Internal Revenue Service

**Employer's Annual Federal
Unemployment (FUTA) Tax Return**
▶ For Paperwork Reduction Act Notice, see page 2.

OMB No. 1545-0028

1990

			T	
	Name (as distinguished from trade name)	Calendar year	FF	
If incorrect, make any necessary change. ▶	Trade name, if any		FD	
			FP	
	Address and ZIP code	Employer identification number	I	
		—	T	

A Did you pay all required contributions to state unemployment funds by the due date of Form 940? (See instructions if none required.) . . . . ☐ Yes ☐ No
  If you checked the "Yes" box, enter the amount of contributions paid to state unemployment funds. . . . . ▶ $ _____
B Are you required to pay contributions to only one state? . . . . ☐ Yes ☐ No
  If you checked the "Yes" box: (1) Enter the name of the state where you are required to pay contributions . . . . ▶ _____
  (2) Enter your state reporting number(s) as shown on state unemployment tax return. ▶ _____
C If any part of wages taxable for FUTA tax is exempt from state unemployment tax, check the box. (See the Specific Instructions on page 4.) . . . . . ☐
  Note: *If you checked the "Yes" boxes in both questions A and B and did not check the box in C above, you may be able to use Form 940-EZ.*
If you will not have to file returns in the future, write "Final" here (see general instruction "Who Must File") and sign the return. ▶ _____

Part I Computation of Taxable Wages (to be completed by all taxpayers)

1	Total payments (including exempt payments) during the calendar year for services of employees	1	
2	Exempt payments. (Explain each exemption shown, attaching additional sheets if necessary.) ▶ _____	Amount paid	
		2	
3	Payments for services of more than $7,000. Enter only the excess over the first $7,000 paid to individual employees not including exempt amounts shown on line 2. Do not use the state wage limitation.	3	
4	Total exempt payments (add lines 2 and 3)	4	
5	Total taxable wages (subtract line 4 from line 1). (If any part is exempt from state contributions, see instructions.) ▶	5	

Part II Tax Due or Refund (Complete if you checked the "Yes" boxes in both questions A and B and did not check the box in C above.)

1	Total FUTA tax. Multiply the wages in Part I, line 5, by .008 and enter here	1	
2	Total FUTA tax deposited for the year, including any overpayment applied from a prior year (from your records) . .	2	
3	Balance due (subtract line 2 from line 1). This should be $100 or less. Pay to IRS . . . . . . ▶	3	
4	Overpayment (subtract line 1 from line 2). Check if it is to be: ☐ Applied to next return, or ☐ Refunded . ▶	4	

Part III Tax Due or Refund (Complete if you checked the "No" box in either question A or B or you checked the box in C above. Also complete Part V.)

1	Gross FUTA tax. Multiply the wages in Part I, line 5, by .062	1	
2	Maximum credit. Multiply the wages in Part I, line 5, by .054	2	
3	Credit allowable: Enter the smaller of the amount in Part V, line 11, or Part III, line 2 . .	3	
4	Total FUTA tax (subtract line 3 from line 1)	4	
5	Total FUTA tax deposited for the year, including any overpayment applied from a prior year (from your records) . .	5	
6	Balance due (subtract line 5 from line 4). This should be $100 or less. Pay to IRS . . . . . ▶	6	
7	Overpayment (subtract line 4 from line 5). Check if it is to be: ☐ Applied to next return, or ☐ Refunded . ▶	7	

Part IV Record of Quarterly Federal Tax Liability for Unemployment Tax (Do not include state liability.)

Quarter	First	Second	Third	Fourth	Total for Year
Liability for quarter					

Part V Computation of Tentative Credit (Complete if you checked the "No" box in either question A or B or you checked the box in C above—see instructions.)

Name of state (1)	State reporting number(s) as shown on employer's state contribution returns (2)	Taxable payroll (as defined in state act) (3)	State experience rate period From— / To— (4)	State experience rate (5)	Contributions if rate had been 5.4% (col. 3 x .054) (6)	Contributions payable at experience rate (col. 3 x col. 5) (7)	Additional credit (col. 6 minus col. 7) If 0 or less, enter 0. (8)	Contributions actually paid to the state (9)
			From— To—					

10 Totals . . . . ▶

11 Total tentative credit (add line 10, columns 8 and 9 only—see instructions for limitations) . . . . ▶

Under penalties of perjury, I declare that I have examined this return, including accompanying schedules and statements, and to the best of my knowledge and belief, it is true, correct, and complete, and that no part of any payment made to a state unemployment fund claimed as a credit was or is to be deducted from the payments to employees.

Signature ▶ _____ Title (Owner, etc.) ▶ _____ Date ▶ _____

Form **940** (1990)

Figure 3.6 940 form. Employer's annual federal unemployment (FUTA) tax return.

DO NOT STAPLE

1 Control number	ꓱꓱꓱꓱꓱ	For Official Use Only ▶ OMB No. 1545-0008					
☐ Kind of Payer ▶		2 941/941E Military 943 ☐ ☐ ☐ CT-1 942 Medicare gov't. emp. ☐ ☐ ☐			3 Employer's state I.D. number		5 Total number of statements
					4		
6 Establishment number		7 Allocated tips			8 Advance EIC payments		
9 Federal income tax withheld		10 Wages, tips, and other compensation			11 Social security tax withheld		
12 Social security wages		13 Social security tips			14 Nonqualified plans		
15 Dependent care benefits		16 Adjusted total social security wages and tips			17 Deferred compensation		
18 Employer's identification number					19 Other EIN used this year		
20 Employer's name					21 Gross annuity, pension, etc. (Form W-2P)		
					23 Taxable amount (Form W-2P)		
					24 Income tax withheld by third-party payer		
22 Employer's address and ZIP code (If available, place label over boxes 18 and 20.)							

Under penalties of perjury, I declare that I have examined this return and accompanying documents, and to the best of my knowledge and belief, they are true, correct, and complete.

Signature ▶ _____ Title ▶ _____ Date ▶ _____

Telephone number (optional) _____

Form **W-3** **Transmittal of Income and Tax Statements** **1990**   Department of the Treasury Internal Revenue Service

Please return this entire page with the accompanying Forms W-2 or W-2P to the Social Security Administration address for your state as listed below. **Household employers filing Forms W-2 for household employees should send the forms to the Albuquerque Data Operations Center.** Note: Extra postage may be necessary if the report you send contains more than a few pages or if the envelope is larger than letter size. Do NOT order forms from the addresses listed below. You may order forms by calling 1-800-424-3676.

If your legal residence, principal place of business, office or agency is located in ▼	Use this address ▼
Alaska, Arizona, California, Colorado, Hawaii, Idaho, Iowa, Minnesota, Missouri, Montana, Nebraska, Nevada, North Dakota, Oregon, South Dakota, Utah, Washington, Wisconsin, Wyoming	Social Security Administration Salinas Data Operations Center Salinas, CA 93911
Alabama, Arkansas, Florida, Georgia, Illinois, Kansas, Louisiana, Mississippi, New Mexico, Oklahoma, South Carolina, Tennessee, Texas	Social Security Administration Albuquerque Data Operations Center Albuquerque, NM 87180
Connecticut, Delaware, District of Columbia, Indiana, Kentucky, Maine, Maryland, Massachusetts, Michigan, New Hampshire, New Jersey, New York, North Carolina, Ohio, Pennsylvania, Rhode Island, Vermont, Virginia, West Virginia	Social Security Administration Wilkes-Barre Data Operations Center Wilkes-Barre, PA 18769
If you have no legal residence or principal place of business in any state	Social Security Administration Wilkes-Barre Data Operations Center Wilkes-Barre, PA 18769

Paperwork Reduction Act Notice.—We ask for this information to carry out the Internal Revenue laws of the United States. We need it to ensure that taxpayers are complying with these laws and to allow us to figure and collect the right amount of tax. You are required to give us this information.

The time needed to complete and file this form will vary depending on individual circumstances.

The estimated average time is 26 minutes. If you have comments concerning the accuracy of this time estimate or suggestions for making this form more simple, we would be happy to hear from you. You can write to the **Internal Revenue Service,** Washington, DC 20224, Attention: IRS Reports Clearance Officer T:FP; or the **Office of Management and Budget,** Paperwork Reduction Project (1545-0008), Washington, DC 20503.

Figure 3.7   W-3 form. Transmittal of income and tax statements.

Internal Organization

So you know how you are going to structure your business and what your tax liability will be. Now you have to give some thought to how you are going to structure your internal operation.

Obviously, if you are going to start small, you are going to do it all. Hopefully you will get some assistance from a bookkeeper, an accountant, and perhaps even an attorney.

If you are going to really jump into this thing, you will be considering hiring people to assist you in various portions of your processing operation. These individuals will be organized into management and staff. Before you rush into hiring people to fill these slots, you need to think about just what the management of your business is going to entail.

Management is a learned skill. Look at how many people are spending enormous amounts of time and money to capture the jewel of the business world—the MBA (Master of Business Administration, for you novices). When you are starting your own manufacturing operation, often you (diamond-in-the-rough) must offer direction and control of the entire operation. Too often, entrepreneur food processors tend to drift with the current, barely getting by from crisis to crisis. They become veteran fire fighters, solving immediate problems but not developing a plan of operations. In effect, they let their business run them—a very interesting management style. This kind of operation is sure to give you ulcers within 3 years of processing your first jar of jelly!

Management involves the creative manipulation of events and people to produce future as well as current profits. It requires both short- and long-term strategies. You must constantly work at strategizing the use of money, material, and manpower to make your company work at its most efficient. Producing 100 cases of jelly an hour instead of 95, with the same amount of manpower, equipment, utility usage, and space expenses, will earn you that much more clear profit.

You must set measurable objectives. You must track how much raw material, how much packaging, and how many man hours it takes to produce so many cases of product. If you don't meet your objectives, find out why. Were the numbers overly ambitious, or is your staff undermotivated? Are you wasting sugar, or is your equipment not set up to handle the grain flow optimally? Keeping tabs on problems while working with set parameters is *good* management.

Production must be closely managed. Timetables must be developed. When must raw materials be on hand? When must new packaging materials be ordered? When must products be shipped? A system of management must be developed whereby authority is delegated to allow for a stable and continuing production pattern. We will discuss this more in depth in Chapter 5.

CHAPTER 4

Raising Capital

Now that you know what you're going to produce and how you are going to set up your company, you have to come up with the dollars to pay for all this. Your friends won't take your new food processing endeavor very seriously until you start writing checks.

You need to make absolutely sure that you know exactly how much money you need and that you have identified all possible financing sources before you start negotiations. Insufficient financing is the *major* cause of small business failure. If you don't include adequate capital (enough to operate over a specific period of time) in your business strategy, you will not get very far. If you are not particularly savvy about business financing, find some professional assistance. There are state, federal, and local agencies available, with highly trained professionals who would be happy to share their knowledge with you (see Appendices A–D). Lack of financial understanding and planning can be devastating to the entrepreneur. You can obtain the wrong kind of financing, over- or underestimate the amount of financing needed (a very common problem), fail to synchronize your funding with all your actual start-up and operating costs, or underestimate the real cost of money.

Before you set out to seek the capital you need, you must figure out exactly what your financial requirements are going to be. Can you obtain enough money from your own family and friends' resources, or will you need debt- or equity-type financing? Be sure to get some financial counseling at this point. It is usually available at little or no cost.

Business Plan

This is the best time to put together your business plan. It will not only focus your marketing strategies, it will help you identify how much money you need and how it will be spent. Banks look much more favorably on business persons who apply for start-up money armed with a strong business plan.

There are hundreds of books, pamphlets, articles, and even software programs designed to help you write a business plan. The following excellent outline was developed by the staff of the University of Colorado Business Advancement Center. Also included at the end of this chapter is a glossary of commonly used terms.

Suggested Outline

Cover Sheet: Name of business, names of principals, address and phone number of business.

Statement of Purpose

Table of Contents
1. The Business
   a. Description of business
   b. Market
   c. Competition
   d. Location of business
   e. Management
   f. Personnel
   g. Application and expected effect of loan (if needed)
   h. Summary
2. Financial Data
   a. Sources and applications of funding
   b. Capital equipment list
   c. Balance sheet

d. Breakeven analysis
e. Income projections (profit and loss statements)
   1) 3-year summary
   2) Detail by month for first year
   3) Detail by quarter for second and third years
   4) Notes of explanation
f. Pro forma cash flow
   1) Detail by month for first year
   2) Detail by quarter for second and third years
   3) Notes of explanation
g. Deviation analysis
h. Historical financial reports for existing business
   1) Balance sheets for past 3 years
   2) Tax returns
3. Supporting Documents
   Personal resumes, job descriptions, personal financial statements, credit reports, letters of reference, letters of intent, copies of leases, contracts, and legal documents, and anything else of relevance to the plan.

Introduction

The business plan is your company's principal sales tool in raising capital. Before risking any capital, investors want to assure themselves that you have thought through your plans carefully, that you know what you are doing, and that you can respond effectively to problems and opportunities. They will insist on seeing your business plan before considering any investment and often will not even meet with entrepreneurs without a prior review of the business plan. Therefore, your business plan must be well prepared and persuasive in conveying the potential of the company it describes. It should address all major issues, yet not be so detailed that it "turns off" the investor–reader. You should try not to have a business plan more than 50 pages long.

The guidelines that follow describe:

1. The necessary sections of a business plan;
2. What should be included in each section and subsection; and
3. Why the information is necessary and where to find it.

Intelligent use of these guidelines should result in a complete professional business plan which makes an orderly presentation of the facts necessary to obtain an investment decision. Common sense should be used in applying the guidelines to develop a business plan for each venture.

Because the guidelines were written to cover a variety of possible ventures, rigid adherence to them is not possible or even desirable for all ventures. For example, a plan for a service business would not require a discussion of manufacturing or product design.

Summary

Most investors do not like to wade immediately through a 40- or 50-page business proposal. Before doing this, they like to read a 1- or 2-page summary of the business plan that highlights its important features and allows them to determine quickly whether or not the venture is of interest. The summary also saves the entrepreneur time since he doesn't have to wait for the investor to read 40–50 pages to express interest.

You should prepare a 1- to 2-page summary of your business plan. It should be a brief, appealing, and accurate presentation of the highlights of your venture and its opportunities.

The Company and Its Founders

You should indicate when the company was formed, what it will do, and what is special or unique about this. Also indicate what in the backgrounds of the entrepreneurs makes them particularly qualified (e.g., unique know-how) to pursue the business opportunity.

Market Opportunity

Identify and explain (briefly) the market opportunity. This explanation should include information on the size and growth rate of the market for the company's product or service and a statement indicating the percentage of that market that will be captured. A brief statement about industry-wide trends is also useful. You might also indicate any plans for the expansion of the initial product line.

Financial Data

You should state your initial and third-year sales and profit goals. You should also state clearly the size and equity investment you want and any long-term loans that you can obtain.

Text

The Company and Its Industry

This section should describe the nature and history of the company and provide some background on its industry. It provides the potential investor with insights that allow him to better understand the projection and estimates presented in subsequent sections.

The Company

Give the date that the venture became a legal entity, indicate whether the business is or will be profit or nonprofit, and exactly how the corporation will be set up (conducted as a separate corporation).

Describe the general business category the company is entering. State specifically why the company is being formed and what opportunities you see for its products, processes, or services. Describe the identification and development of the business opportunity and the involvements or the principals in that development.

A personal financial statement should be included for all principals. Box 4.1 is an example of a personal financial statement.

Discussion of Industry

Present the current status and prospects for the industry in which the proposed business will operate.

Discuss any new products or developments, new markets and customers, new requirements, new companies, and any other trends and factors that could affect the venture's business positively or negatively. Identify the source of all information used to describe industry trends.

BOX 4.1
PERSONAL FINANCIAL STATEMENT
_____ _____ 19___

Assets

Cash $ _____

Savings accounts _____

Stocks, bonds, other securities _____

Accounts/notes receivable _____

Life insurance cash value _____

Rebates/refunds _____

Autos/other vehicles _____

Real estate _____

Vested pension plan/retirement accounts _____

Other assets _____

Total assets $ _____

Liabilities

Accounts payable $ _____

Contracts payable _____

Notes payable _____

Taxes _____

Real estate loans _____

Other liabilities _____

Total liabilities $ _____

Total Assets $ _____

Less Total Liabilities ⁻$ _____

Net Worth $ _____

Products or Services

The potential investor will be vitally interested in exactly what you are going to sell, what kind of product protection you have, and the opportunities and possible drawbacks to your product or service. This section deals with these questions.

Description

Describe in detail the products or services to be sold. Discuss the application or function for the product or service that you will offer. Describe the primary end use as well as any significant secondary applications. Highlight any differences between what is currently on the market and what you will offer.

Define the present state of development of the product or service. For products, provide a summary of the functional specifications. Include photographs when available.

Proprietary Position

Describe any patents, trade secrets, or other proprietary features. Attach copies of any patents applied for or granted. Discuss any headstart that you might have that would enable you to achieve a favored or entrenched position.

Potential

Describe any features of your product or service that may give it an advantage over the competition. Discuss any opportunities for the expansion of the product line or the development of related products or services. Emphasize your opportunities and explain how you will take advantage of them.

Discuss any product disadvantages or the possibilities of rapid obsolescence because of technological or styling changes or marketing fads.

Market Research and Evaluation

To be an attractive investment, a company should be selling to a market that is large and growing—where a small market share can be a significant sales volume. The company's competition should be profitable but not so strong as to overwhelm you.

The purpose of this section is to present sufficient facts to convince the reader that the product or service has a substantial market and can achieve sales in the face of the competition.

Customers

Discuss who are the customers for the anticipated application of the product or service. Classify potential customers into relatively homogeneous groups (major market segment) having common, identifiable characteristics. For example, an automotive part might be sold to *manufacturers* and to *parts distributors* supplying the replacement market.

Who and where are the major purchasers for the product or service in each market segment? What are the bases of their purchase decisions: price, quality, service, personal contact, political pressures?

List any potential customers who have expressed an interest in the product or service and indicate why. List any potential customers who have shown no interest in the proposed product or service and explain why this is so. Explain what you will do to overcome negative customer reaction.

Market Size and Trends

What is the size of the current *total* market for the product or service offered? This market size should be determined from available data or the purchases of potential customers in each major market segment. Describe the size of the total market in both units and dollars. If you intend to sell regionally, show the regional market size. Indicate the sources of data and methods used to establish current market size. State also the credentials of people doing market research.

Describe the potential annual growth of the total market for your product or service for each major customer group. Total market projections should be made for at least 3 future years. Discuss the major factors affecting market growth (industry trends, socioeconomic trends, government policy, population shifts) and review previous trends of the market. Any differences between past and projected annual growth rates should be explained. Indicate the sources of all data and methods used to make projections.

Competition

Make a realistic assessment of the strengths and weaknesses of competitive products and services and name the companies that supply them. State data sources used to determine products and strength of competition.

Compare competing products or services on the basis of price, performance, service, warranties, and other pertinent features. A table can be an effective way of presenting these data. Present a short discussion of the current advantages and disadvantages of competing products and services and say why they are not meeting customer needs. Indicate any knowledge of competitors' actions that could lead you to new or improved products and an advantageous position.

Review the strengths and weaknesses of the competing companies. Determine and discuss the share of the market of each competitor company—sales, distribution, and production capabilities. Review also the profitability of competitors and their profit trends. Who is the pricing leader? The quality leader? Discuss why any companies have entered or dropped out of the market in recent years.

Discuss your three or four key competitors and why the customer buys from them. From what you know about their operations, explain why you think you can capture a share of their business. Discuss what makes you think it will be easy or difficult to compete with them.

Estimated Market Share and Sales

Describe what it is about your product or service that will make it saleable in the face of current and potential competition.

Identify any major first-year customers who are willing to make purchase commitments. Indicate the extent of those commitments and why they were made. Discuss which customers could be major purchasers in subsequent years and why.

Based on your assessment of the advantages of your product or service, the market size and trends, customers, and the competition and their products, estimate the share of the market that you will acquire in each of the next 3 years. The growth of sales and the company's estimated market share should be related to the growth

TABLE 4.1
Estimated Market Share

Estimate	First year (quarters)				Year			
	1st	2nd	3rd	4th	2	3	4	5
Total market (dollars)	—	—	—	—	—	—	—	—
Market share (%)	—	—	—	—	—	—	—	—
Sales (dollars)	—	—	—	—	—	—	—	—

of the industry and customers and the strengths and weaknesses of competitors. The data can best be presented in tabular form as shown in Table 4.1. The assumptions used to estimate market share and sales should be clearly stated.

Ongoing Market Evaluation

Explain how you will continue to evaluate your target markets so as to assess customer needs and guide product improvement programs and new-product programs, plan for expansions of your production facility, and guide product/service pricing.

Marketing Plan

The marketing plan should detail the overall marketing strategy, sales and service policies, and pricing, distribution, and advertising strategies that will be used to achieve the estimated market share and sales projections. The marketing plan should describe what is to be done, *how* it will be done, and *who* will do it. The plan should be prepared by the marketer of the management with assistance from consultants as may be required.

Overall Marketing Strategy

Describe the general marketing philosophy and strategy of the company that develops from the market research and evaluation. This should include a discussion of the following questions.

What kinds of customer groups will be targeted for initial intensive selling effort? What customer groups will be targeted for later selling efforts? What features of the product or service (e.g., quality, price, delivery, warranty) will be emphasized to generate sales? Are there any innovative or unusual marketing concepts that will enhance customer acceptance (e.g., leasing where only sales were previously attempted)?

Indicate whether the product or service will initially be introduced nationally or on a regional level. If on a regional basis, explain why and indicate any plans for extending sales to other sections of the country. Discuss any sectional trends and what can be done to promote sales out of season.

Describe any plans to obtain government contracts as means of supporting manufacturing or product development costs and overhead.

Pricing

The pricing policy is one of the more important decisions you will have to make. The "price must be right" to penetrate the market, maintain a market position, and produce profits.

Discuss the prices to be charged for your product and service and compare your pricing policy with those of your major competitors. Discuss the gross profit margin between manufacturing and ultimate sales costs. Indicate whether this margin is large enough to allow for distribution and sales, warranty, service, amortization of development and equipment costs, and price competition and still allow you a profit.

Explain how the price you set will enable you to (a) Get the product or service accepted; (b) Maintain and desirably increase your market share in the face of competition; and (c) Produce profits.

Justify any price increases over competitive items on the basis of newness, quality, warranty, and service.

If a price lower than your competition's is to be charged, explain how you will do this and maintain profitability—for example, greater effectiveness in manufacturing and distributing the product, lower labor costs, lower overhead, or lower material costs.

Discuss the relationship of price, market share, and profits. For example, a higher price may reduce volume but result in a higher gross profit. Describe any discount allowance for prompt payment or volume purchases.

Sales Tactics

Describe the methods that will be used to make sales and distribute the product or service. Will the company use its own sales force? Sales representatives? Distributors? Are there ready-made manufacturer's organizations already selling related products that can be used? Describe both the initial plans and the longer-range plans for a sales force. Discuss the margins to be given to retailers, wholesalers, and salesmen and compare them to those given by your competition.

If distributors or sales representatives are to be used describe how they have been selected, when they will start to represent you, and the areas they will cover. Show a table that indicates the build-up of dealers and representatives by month and the expected sales to be made by each dealer. Describe any special policies regarding discounts, exclusive distribution rights, etc.

If a direct-sales force is to be used, indicate how it will be structured and at what rate it will be built up. If it is to replace a dealer or representative organization indicate when and how. Show the sales expected per salesperson per year and what commission incentive and/or salary the salespeople are slated to receive.

If original equipment manufacturer (OEM) or government contracts are expected or essential, discuss how, why, and when these will be obtained.

Present, as an exhibit, a selling schedule and a sales budget that includes all marketing, promotion, and service costs. This sales-expense exhibit should also indicate when sales will commence and the lapse between a sale and a delivery.

Service and Warranty Policies

If your company will offer a product that will require service and warranties, indicate the importance of these to the customer's purchasing decision and discuss your method of handling service problems. Describe the kind and term of any warranties to be offered, whether service will be handled by company service representatives, agencies, dealers, and distributors, or factory return. Indicate the proposed charge for service calls and whether service will be a profitable or a break-even operation. Compare your service and warranty policies and practices with those of your principal competitors and indicate what kinds of service manuals will be prepared.

Advertising and Promotion

Describe the approaches the company will use to bring its product to the attention of prospective purchasers. For OEM and industrial products indicate the plans for trade-show participation, trade-magazine advertisements, direct mailings, preparation of product sheets and promotional literature, and use of advertising agencies. For consumer products indicate what kind of advertising and promotional campaign is contemplated to introduce the product and what kinds of sales aids will be provided to dealers. The schedule and cost of promotion and advertising should be presented. If advertising will be a significant part of company expenses, an exhibit showing how and when these costs will be incurred should be included.

Design and Development Plans

If the product, process, or service of the proposed venture requires any design and development before it is ready to be placed on the market, the nature and extent of this work should be fully discussed. The investor will want to know the extent and nature of any design and development and the costs and time required to achieve a marketable product. Such design and development might be the engineering work necessary to convert a laboratory prototype to a finished product, or the design of special tooling, or the work of an industrial designer to make a product more attractive and saleable, or the identification and organization of manpower, equipment, and special techniques to implement a service business (e.g., the equipment, new computer software, and skills required for computerized credit checking).

Development Status and Tasks

Describe the current status of the product or service and explain what remains to be done to make it marketable. Describe, briefly, the competence or expertise that your company has or can acquire to complete this development. Indicate the type and extent of technical assistance that will be required and state who will supervise this activity within your organization and his or her experience in related development work.

Difficulties and Risks

Identify any major anticipated design and development problems and approaches to their solution. Discuss their possible effect on the schedule and cost of design and development and the time of market introduction.

Product Improvement and New Products

In addition to describing the development of the initial products, discuss any ongoing design and development work that is planned to keep your product or service competitive and develop new related products that can be sold to the same group of customers.

Costs

Present and discuss a design and development budget. The costs should include labor, materials, consulting fees, etc. Miscalculations are often made about design and development costs and this can have a serious impact on cash-flow projections. Accordingly, consider and perhaps show a 10–20% cost contingency. This cost data will become an integral part of the financial plan.

Manufacturing and Operations Plan

The manufacturing and operations plan should describe the kind of facilities, plant location, space requirements, capital equipment, and labor force (part and full time) that are required to provide the company's product or service. For a manufacturing business, stress should also be given to the production process that will be used, to inventory control, purchasing, and production control, and to """make or buy decisions" (i.e., which parts of the product will be purchased and which operations will be performed by your work force). A service business may require particular attention and focus on an appropriate location and an ability to minimize overhead, lease the required equipment, and obtain competitive productivity from a skilled or trained labor force.

The discussion guidelines given below are general enough to cover both product and service businesses. Only those that are relevant to your venture, be it product or service, should be addressed in your business plan.

Geographical Location

Describe the planned geographical location of the business and discuss any advantages or disadvantages of the site location in terms of wage rates, labor unionization, labor availability, closeness to customers or suppliers, access to transportation, state and local taxes and laws, utilities, and zoning. For a service business, proximity to customers is a "must." Describe your approach to overcoming any problems associated with location.

Facilities and Improvements

Describe the facilities required to start and conduct the company's business. Indicate the requirements for plant and office space, storage and land areas, machinery, special tooling, and other capital equipment, and utilities. Discuss any facilities currently owned or leased that could be used for the proposed venture.

Describe how and when initial plant space and equipment will be expanded to the capacities required by future sales projections. Discuss any plans to improve or add to existing plant space or move the facility. Explain future equipment needs and indicate the timing and cost of such acquisitions. A 3-year planning period should be used for these projections.

Strategy and Plans

Describe the manufacturing processes involved in your product's production and any decisions with respect to subcontracting of component parts rather than complete in-house manufacture. The "make or buy" strategy adopted should be determined by consideration of inventory financing, available labor skills, and other nontechnical questions as well as purely production, cost, and capability issues (your company might operate as a labor-intensive assembly plant and purchase basic parts and subassemblies). Justify your proposed "make or buy" policy. Discuss any surveys of potential subcontractors and suppliers and who these are likely to be.

Present a production or operations plan that shows cost–volume information at various sales levels of operation with full breakdowns of applicable material, labor, purchased component, and factory burden. Discuss the inventory required at various sales levels. These data will be incorporated into cash-flow projections. The operations plan should also discuss the build-up in the labor force and relate the added labor hours to increased output. Explain how any seasonal production loads will be handled without severe dislocation, for example, by building to inventory or part-time help in peak periods. If there are daily shift-to-shift variations in the labor force (for a service business) discuss them and how they will be handled.

Briefly, describe your approach to quality control, production control, and inventory control. Explain what quality control and inspection procedures the company will use to minimize service problems and associated customer dissatisfaction.

Discuss how you will organize and operate your purchasing function to ensure that adequate materials are on hand for production, that the best price has been obtained, and that raw materials and in-process inventory, and hence, working capital, have been minimized.

Labor Force

Exclusive of management functions (discussed later), does the local labor force have the necessary skills in sufficient quantity and quality (lack of absenteeism, productivity) to manufacture the product or supply the services of the proposed company? If the skills of the labor force are inadequate to meet the needs of the company, describe the kinds of training that you will use to upgrade skills. Discuss whether the new business can offer such training and still offer a competitive product both in the short term (first year) and in the longer term (2–5 years).

Management Team

The management team is the key to turning a good idea into a successful business. Investors look for a committed management team with a proper balance of technical, managerial, and business skills and experience in doing what is proposed.

Accordingly, this section of the business plan will be of primary interest to potential investors and will significantly influence their investment decisions. It should include a description of the key management personnel and their primary duties, the organizational structure, the Board of Directors, and any management training that will be required.

Organization

Present in tabular form the key management roles in the company and name the individual who will fill each position.

Discuss any experience where the management team has worked together that indicates how their skills complement each other and result in an effective entrepreneurial–management team.

If any key individuals will not be on board at the start of the venture, indicate when they will join the company.

In a new business, it may not be possible to fill each executive role with a full-time person without excessively burdening the overhead of the venture. One solution is to use part-time specialists or consultants to perform some functions. If this is your plan, discuss it and indicate who will be used and when they will be replaced by full-time staff members.

If the company is of sufficient size, an organizational chart can be appended as an exhibit.

Key Management Personnel

Describe the exact duties and responsibilities of each of the key members of the management team. Include a brief (3- or 4-sentence) statement of the career highlights of each individual that focuses on accomplishments demonstrating the person's ability to perform in the assigned role.

Complete resumes for each key management member should be included as an exhibit to the business plan. These resumes should stress the training, experience, and accomplishments of each manager in performing functions similar to his or her role in the venture. Accomplishments should be discussed in such concrete terms as profit improvement, labor management, manufacturing or technical achievements, ability to meet budgets and schedules, and community organization. Where possible it should be noted who can attest to accomplishments and what recognition or rewards were received, for example, pay increases, promotions, etc. A sample resume format is attached (see Box 4.2).

Management Compensation and Ownership

The likelihood of obtaining financing is small when the founding management team is not prepared to accept initial modest salaries. If the founders demand substantial salaries, the potential

BOX 4.2
SAMPLE MANAGEMENT RESUME

John Jones—Vice President, Marketing

Age: 40   Health: Excellent

Married, 1 Child   Height/Weight: 6 ft, 170 lb.

Summary: Ten years of marketing experience in the leisure
                       products industry. Both product manager as
                       well as sales manager with profit and loss
                       responsibility for a complete product line of
                       tents.

Experience
1962–1969   *Leisure Corp., Brooklyn, NY*
                       Marketing Manager for entire line of tents with
                       total responsibility for profitability. Functions
                       include sales planning, advertising, and pub-
                       lications. U.S. operations started from scratch
                       to present $6 million/year, always at a profit.

December, 1954 to   *American Systems, Brooklyn, NY*
September, 1962   Sales Manager, accounting equipment. Super-
                       vised 5 salesmen. $2 million/year.

Education   University of Illinois—B.A. in Liberal Arts, 1954.

Professional   American Society of Managers, Society of
Associations   Mercantile Merchandisers, American Market-
                       ing Federation, Two Million Dollar Salesman's
                       Club

References   Available upon request

investor will conclude that their psychological commitment to the venture is less than it should be.

State the salary that is to be paid to each key person and compare it to the salary recieved at his or her last independent job. Set forth the stock ownership planned for key personnel, the amount of their equity investment (if any), and any performance-dependent stock-option or bonus plans that are contemplated.

Board of Directors

By establishing an effective Board of Directors, management can obtain (1) the participation of local residents to ensure that the business is properly responsive to community needs and effectively taps local resources, and (2) advice and assistance in dealing with customers and suppliers.

Discuss the company's philosophy as to the size and composition of the Board. Identify any proposed board members and include a 1- or 2-sentence statement of each member's background that shows what he or she can bring to the company. Resumes for each board member should be included as an exhibit to the business plan.

Management Assistance and Training Needs

Describe, candidly, the strengths and weaknesses of your management team and Board of Directors. Discuss the kind, extent, and timing of any *management* training that will be required to overcome the weaknesses and obtain effective venture operation.

Discuss also the need for technical and management assistance during the first 3 years of your venture. Be as specific as you can as to the kind, extent, and cost of such assistance and how it will be obtained.

Supporting Professional Services

State the legal (including patent), accounting, advertising, and banking organizations that you have selected for your venture. Capable, reputable, and well-known supporting service organizations (Table 4.2) can not only provide significant direct, professional assistance, but can also add to the credibility of your venture. In addition, properly selected professional organizations can help you establish good contacts in the business community, identify potential investors, and secure financing.

TABLE 4.2
Professional Assistance Available

Adviser

Accountant

Type of assistance: Can set up a pattern of bookkeeping that is easy for the owner to follow daily and for the accountant to work with at audit or tax time. Helps set up systems for the control of cash and handling of funds and can suggest simple equipment like cash registers, multiple-copy sales checks, and other forms.

How to find it: Bankers and lawyers often know accountants who are willing to work with small businesses. Accountants are listed in the Yellow Pages. The entrepreneur should confer with several accountants and check their experience and references before deciding on one. Fees are often based on hourly rates and vary with the complexity and extent of the service. Fees should be negotiated in advance.

Attorney

Type of assistance: Can help choose a form of business, drawing up partnership and incorporating agreements, make sure papers are properly filed with city, county, and state governments, interpret contracts and leases, arbitrate disputes within the business and for the business against others, and consult when the business owner is unsure of legal rights and obligations.

How to find it: Lawyers may be located through friends, other business owners, suppliers, consultants, trade associations, or listings in the Yellow Pages. In most counties, local bar association referral services can arrange for a business person in need of legal counsel to meet with a practicing attorney in the area. The initial consultation implies no further obligation.

Banker

Type of assistance: Has financial knowledge (loans, separate checking accounts for the business, other funding or bank services such as billing service and credit systems), is familiar with the community, may suggest individuals and other institutions that can be helpful.

(continued)

TABLE 4.2 (*continued*)

Adviser

Banker (*continued*)

How to find it: A banker might be contacted where the business owner has a personal bank account or near the business location for convenience. It is often advisable to establish a continuing relationship, keeping the banker informed of the progress of the business.

Insurance agent or broker

Type of assistance: Will evaluate insurance needs and set up packages to cover specific types of businesses. May be either an independent (dealing with several insurance companies) or a direct writer (employed by and writing policies for one company).

How to find it: The business operator should talk with several agents, compare the coverage and costs of the insurance they offer, and select the program best suited to the company's needs, comprehensively and economically. Agents require complete data on business operations and must be continuously apprised of changes affecting insurance coverage. Agents and brokers are listed in the Yellow Pages.

Management and marketing consultant

Type of assistance: If specializing in small business, can help new business people determine and juggle the many facets of starting — product determination, advertising, inventory, security, filing, hiring, pricing — hidden details that a new entrepreneur may not think of. Has access to other sources of information and contacts with lawyers, accountants, and advertising agencies.

How to find it: Consultants are listed in the Yellow Pages and can be found by talking to friends and others in the business. The Small Business Administration sometimes has suggestions and has its own SCORE (Service Corps of Retired Executives) volunteers who counsel business owners and charge only their out-of-pocket expenses. Consultants generally charge on an hourly, daily, or weekly basis or on a monthly "retainer."

Overall Schedule

A schedule that shows the timing and interrelationship of the major events necessary to launch the venture and realize its objectives is an essential part of a business plan. In addition to being a planning aid and showing deadlines critical to a venture's success, a well-prepared schedule can be an extremely effective sales tool in raising money from potential investors. If properly prepared and realistic, it demonstrates the ability of the management team to plan for venture growth in a way that recognizes obstacles and minimizes investor risk.

Prepare, as a part of this section, a month-by-month schedule that shows the timing of such activities as product development, market planning, sales programs, and production and operations. Sufficient detail should be included to show the timing of the primary tasks required to accomplish an activity.

Show, on the schedule, the deadlines or milestones critical to the venture's success. Events such as the following should be included.

- Incorporation of the venture
- Completion of design and development
- Completion of prototypes (a key date—its achievement is a tangible measure of the company's ability to perform)
- Product display at trade shows
- Ordering of materials in production quantities
- Start of production or operation (another key date because it is related to the production of income)
- First orders received
- First sales and deliveries (a date of maximum interest because it relates directly to the company's credibility and need for capital)
- Payment of first accounts receivable (cash in)

The schedule should also show the following and their relation to the development of the business.

- Number of management personnel
- Number of production and operations personnel
- Additions to plant or equipment

Discuss, in a general way, the activities most likely to cause a schedule slippage and what steps you would take to correct such slippages. Discuss the impact of schedule slippages on the venture's operation, especially its potential viability and capital needs. Keep in mind that the time to do things tends to be underestimated even more than financing requirements. So be realistic about your schedule.

Critical Risks and Assumptions

The development of a business has risks and problems and the business plan invariably contains some implicit assumptions about them. The discovery of any unstated negative factors by potential investors can undermine the credibility of the venture and endanger its financing.

Accordingly, identify and discuss the critical assumptions in the business plan and the major problems that you think you will have to solve to develop the venture. This should include a description of the risks and critical assumptions relating to your industry, your company and its personnel, and your product's market appeal as well as the timing and financing of your start-up.

Among the problem areas that may require discussion are:

- Reliability of sales projections (e.g., market does not develop as fast as predicted)
- Any potentially unfavorable industry-wide trends
- Manufacturing at target costs
- Ability of competitors to underprice or obsolete your product
- Innovation and development required to stay competitive
- Meeting the venture development schedule
- Availability of trained labor
- Procurement of parts or raw materials
- Needs for and timing of initial and additional financing

This list is not meant to be complete but only indicative of the kinds of risks and assumptions that might be discussed.

Indicate which business plan assumptions or potential problems are *most critical* to the success of the venture. Describe your plans for minimizing the impact of unfavorable developments in each area on the success of your venture.

Community Benefits

The proposed venture should be an instrument of community and human development as well as economic development, and it should be responsive to the expressed desires of the community.

Describe and discuss the potential economic and noneconomic benefits to members of the community that could result from the formation of the proposed venture.

Some of the benefits that may merit discussion are listed in the next three sections.

Economic

- Number of jobs generated in each of the first 3 years of the venture
- Number and kind of new employment opportunities for previously unemployed or underemployed individuals
- Number of skilled and higher-paying jobs
- Ownership and control of venture assets by community residents
- Purchase of goods and services from local suppliers

Human Development

- New technical skills development and associated career opportunities for community residents
- Management development and training
- Employment of unique skills within the community that are now unused

Community Development

- Development of community's physical assets
- Improved perception of Community Development Council (CDC) responsiveness and their role in the community
- Provision of needed, but unsupplied, services or products to community
- Improvements in the living environment
- Community support, participation, and pride in venture
- Development of community-owned economic structure and decreased absentee business ownership

Describe any compromises or time lags in venture profitability that may result from trying to achieve some or all of the kinds of benefits cited above. Any such compromises or lags in profitability should be justified in the context of all the benefits achieved and the role of the venture in a total, planned program of economic, human, and community development.

The Financial Plan

The financial plan is basic to the evaluation of an investment opportunity and should represent the entrepreneur's best estimates of future operations. Its purpose is to indicate the venture's potential and the timetable for financial viability. It can also serve as an operating plan for financial management of the venture by providing management with the information for planning and control of fund flows.

In developing the financial plans, five basic exhibits must be prepared:

1. Profit and loss forecasts for 3 years
2. Cash-flow projections for 3 years
3. Pro forma balance sheets for 3 years
4. Sources of capital funds (initial and projected)
5. Historic financial data for existing business

Sample forms for preparing these have been provided as Boxes 4.3–4.7. It is recommended that the venture's financial and marketing personnel prepare them with assistance from accountants and venture packagers as required.

In addition to these five basic financial exhibits, a break-even chart should be presented that shows the level of first-year production that is required to cover *all* operating costs.

Profit and Loss Forecast

The preparation of a pro forma income statement (Box 4.3) is the planning-for-profit part of financial management. Crucial to the earnings forecasts—as well as other projections—is the sales forecast. The methods for developing sales forecasts have been described previously in the section on market research and evaluation, and the sales data projected should be used here.

Once the sales forecasts are in hand, production (or operations for a service business) should be budgeted. There must be a

BOX 4.3
PROJECTED PROFIT AND LOSS STATEMENT

	Month 1	Month 2	Month 3	Month 4	Month 5	Month 6	Month 7	Month 8	Month 9	Month 10	Month 11	Month 12
Total Net Sales												
Cost of Sales												
Gross Profit												
Controllable Expenses												
Salaries												
Payroll taxes												
Security												
Advertising												
Automobile												
Dues and subscriptions												
Legal and accounting												
Office supplies												
Telephone												
Utilities												

Miscellaneous														
Total Controllable Expenses														
Fixed Expenses														
Depreciation														
Insurance														
Rent														
Taxes and licenses														
Loan payments														
Total Fixed Expenses														
Total Expenses														
Net Profit (Loss) (before taxes)														

determination of the level of production or operation that is required to meet the sales forecasts and fulfill inventory requirements. The material, labor, service, and equipment requirements must be developed and translated into cost data. A separation of the fixed and variable elements of these costs is desirable, and the effect of sales volume on inventory, equipment acquisitions, and manufacturing costs should be taken into account. The development of these cost data were described in more detail in the section on the manufacturing and operations plan.

Sales expense should include the costs of selling and distribution, storage, discounts, advertising, and promotion. General and administrative expense should include management salaries, secretarial costs, and legal and accounting expenses. Manufacturing or operations overhead includes rent, utilities, fringe benefits, telephone, etc.

Earnings projections should be prepared monthly in the first year of operation and quarterly for the second and third years.

In addition to serving as a basis for planning, the projected income statements can be used for operating control functions. Through comparisons with actual operating sales and profit information, the operating status of the venture can be determined relative to the objectives that have been set in the plan. This type of analysis can be used by management to indicate critical factors which need attention and can indicate the need for a reassessment of the underlying assumptions used to develop the projections.

Discussion of assumptions Because of the importance of profit and loss projections as an indication of the potential financial feasibility of any new venture to potential investors, it is extremely important that the assumptions made in their preparation be fully explained and documented. If these statements are to be useful they must represent management's realistic assessment and best estimates of probable operating results. Sales or operational cost projections that are either too conservative or too optimistic have little value as aids to policy formulation and decision making. *Thinking about assumptions before startup is useful for identifying issues which require consideration before they turn into major problems.*

As well as explanations for the projected sales growth, include any assumptions made about cost of sales expenses, such as materials purchases, direct labor, manufacturing overhead, etc., and general and administrative expenses. These assumptions should be attached to the earnings projections.

Risks and sensitivity Once the income statements have been prepared, discuss the major risks that could prevent those goals from being attained and the sensitivity of profits to these risks.

This discussion should reflect the entrepreneur's thinking about some of the risks that might be encountered in the firm itself, the industry, and the environment. This should include things as different as the effect of a 20% reduction in sales projections and the impact of learning-curve requirements for management and nonmanagement employees that will affect the level of productivity over time.

Pro Forma Cash-Flow Analysis

For a new venture the cash-flow forecast can be more important than the forecasts of profits because it details the amount and timing of expected cash inflows and outflows. Usually the level of profits, particularly during the start-up years of a venture, will not be sufficient to finance operating asset needs. Moreover, cash inflows do not match outflows on a short-term basis. The cash-flow forecast will indicate these conditions and enable management to plan cash needs.

Given a level of projected sales and capital expenditures over a specific period, the cash forecast will highlight the need for additional financing and indicate peak requirements for working capital. Management must decide how this additional financing is to be obtained, on what terms, and how it is to be repaid. This information becomes part of the final cash-flow forecast.

If the venture is in a seasonal or cyclical industry or is in an industry in which suppliers require a new firm to pay cash, or if inventory build-up occurs before the product can be sold for revenues, this cash forecast is crucial to the continuing solvency of the business. A detailed cash-flow forecast which is understood and used by management can enable them to direct their attention to operating problems without distractions caused by periodic crises which should have been anticipated. Cash-flow projections should be made for each month of the fiscal year of operation and quarterly for the second and third years.

BOX 4.4
CASH FLOW PROJECTIONS

	Start-up or prior to loan	Month 1	Month 2	Month 3	Month 4	Month 5	Month 6	Month 7	Month 8	Month 9	Month 10	Month 11	Month 12	Total
Cash (beginning of month)														
Cash on hand														
Cash in bank														
Cash in investments														
Total Cash														
Income (during month)														
Cash sales														
Credit sales payments														
Investment income														
Loans														
Other cash income														
Total income														
Total Cash and Income														

Expenses (during month)

Inventory or new material												
Wages (including owner's)												
Taxes												
Equipment expense												
Overhead												
Selling expense												
Transportation												
Loan repayment												
Other case expenses												
Total expenses												
Cash flow excess (end of month)												
Cash flow cumulative (monthly)												

Discussion of assumptions   This should include assumptions made on timing of collection of receivables, trade discounts given, terms of payments to vendors, planned salary and wage increases, anticipated increases in other operating expenses, seasonality characteristics of the business as they affect inventory requirements, and capital equipment purchases. As with the sales and income projections it is also important that these assumptions represent management's best estimates. These assumptions should be attached to the projected cash flows (Box 4.4).

Cash-flow sensitivity   Once the cash flow has been completed, discuss the implications for funds needs that possible changes in some of the crucial assumptions would have. This is designed to enable the entrepreneurial team to test the sensitivity of the cash budget to a variety of assumptions about business factors and to view a wider range of possible outcomes. Investors are vitally interested in this because it helps them estimate the possibility that you will need more cash sooner than planned.

Pro Forma Balance Sheet

The balance sheet (Box 4.5) is used to detail the assets required to support the projected level of operations indicated in the income projections and, through liabilities, how these assets are to be financed. And every accounting transaction can be recorded in terms of its effect on the balance sheet. Investors look to the projected balance sheets to determine debt-to-equity ratios, working capital current ratios, inventory turnover, etc.

In forecasting balance sheet, it will be necessary to project inventory levels, capital expenditures, and incurrence of debt in addition to the other forecasting data described above. Pro forma balance sheets should be prepared at start-up, quarterly for the first year, and at the end of each of the first 3 years of operation.

Discussion of assumptions   Discuss any new major assumptions underlying the preparation of these statements.

Break-even Chart

A break-even chart (Figure 4.1) is a way of determining the level of sales or production at which sales will cover all costs. This

BOX 4.5
BALANCE SHEET
_____   _____ , 19 ___

	Year 1	Year 2	Year 3
Current Assets			
Cash	$ _____	$ _____	$ _____
Accounts receivable	_____	_____	_____
Inventory	_____	_____	_____
Fixed Assets			
Real estate	_____	_____	_____
Fixtures and equipment	_____	_____	_____
Vehicles	_____	_____	_____
Other Assets			
License	_____	_____	_____
Goodwill	_____	_____	_____
Total Assets	$ _____	$ _____	$ _____
Current Liabilities			
Notes payable (due within 1 year)	$ _____	$ _____	$ _____
Accounts payable	_____	_____	_____
Accrued expenses	_____	_____	_____
Taxes owed	_____	_____	_____
Long-Term Liabilities			
Notes payable	_____	_____	_____
(due after 1 year)			
Other	_____	_____	_____
Total liabilities	$ _____	$ _____	$ _____
Net worth (Assets minus liabilities)	$ _____	$ _____	$ _____

Total Liabilities Plus Net
Worth Should Equal Assets

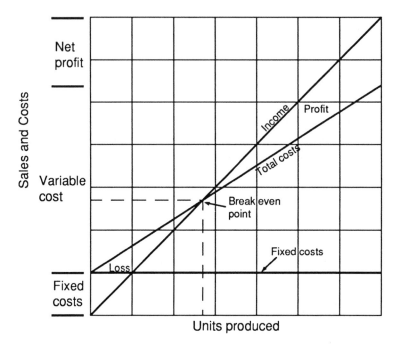

Figure 4.1   Sample break-even chart.

includes those costs that vary with production level (manufacturing labor, material, sales costs) and those that do not change with production level (rent, interest charges, executive salaries, etc.). The sales level that just covers all costs is the minimum sales objective for your venture.

It is very useful for the investor and the management to know what the break-even point is and whether it will be easy or difficult to attain. You should prepare a break-even chart and discuss how the break-even point might be lowered in case you start to fall short of your sales projections. You should also discuss the effect of lower production quantities on the cost of production.

Historic Financial Data for Existing Business

Balance sheets, income statements, and tax returns for the past 3 years should be included for the investor's review along with any pertinent comments. A listing of all capital equipment should also be included.

Proposed Financing

This section is to be devoted to a discussion of the current and proposed capital structure of the venture and to a summary of management's conclusions about the timing and probable sources of funds to meet peak cash requirements. Preparation of this section should be structured so that the following issues are covered:

- Identification of the initial equity investors by name, amount invested, and shares received, and at what cost
- Initial long-term debt, interest rate, repayment terms, and sources
- Description of the type of funding requested
- Description of how the capital funds will be allocated to the various business operations. Approximately how will the funds be used—working capital, equipment purchases, debt repayment (if any)—to cover projected operating losses, etc?
- Based on the cash-flow forecast, management's conclusions about the timing of peak cash needs and how they plan to meet these requirements. For example, securing a line of credit with a local bank, taking on additional long-term debt, attracting new equity investors, factoring receivables, or any combination of these.
- Describe any plans for distributing all or a portion of the stock of the company to the residents of the community. Give the estimated timing and amounts of such distributions.

Two sample charts have been provided as Boxes 4.6 and 4.7 to display initial projected amounts, timing, terms, and sources of (1) initial capital, and (2) capital requirements projected for 5 years. If letters of credit or commitments from bankers or vendors have been received, please attach copies.

BOX 4.6
INITIAL PROPOSED CAPITAL STRUCTURE

Equity

    Owners   _____

    Others   _____

      Total   _____

Debt (Terms)

  SBA   _____

  Bank   _____

  Other (specify)   _____

    Total   _____

Total Debt and Equity   _____

BOX 4.7
PROJECTED CAPITAL REQUIREMENTS

Source	1st Year	2nd Year	3rd Year	4th Year	5th Year
Owner's equity	_____	_____	_____	_____	_____
Bank	_____	_____	_____	_____	_____
Long-term	_____	_____	_____	_____	_____
Short-term	_____	_____	_____	_____	_____
SBA	_____	_____	_____	_____	_____
Other (specify)	_____	_____	_____	_____	_____

Financial Plan

If you are not quite ready to prepare a complete business plan, the following are some simple steps to help you plan your money needs:

1. List exactly what you need the money for: facility, equipment, operating expenses (budget for at least 1 year), salaries.
2. Estimate a dollar figure for each item identified above for the first year of operation (estimate high). For example:

	Annual Expenditure
Facility	$36,000 (rent)
Equipment	150,000 (lease)
Packaging material	100,000
Raw materials	250,000
Salaries	140,000 (5 staff plus self)
Utilities	12,000

3. Plan for how and when you are going to repay the money. Obviously, you are looking for the cheapest possible financing, but it is important to shop around for the longest terms even if the cost of a long-term loan is higher than that of a short-term loan (and it usually will be). It is advantageous for a new business to have as long as possible to repay its initial financing. You will need some time to start generating profits and the long-term package will make your payments smaller during your initial "lean" period. When you become more established, short-term loans, with lower interest rates, will become more attractive because you can repay them as inventory is sold.
4. Decide whether you can afford the cost of the money. Cost of money is the dollar difference between the actual amount of money you receive from the lender and the amount you will pay back in fees and interest. The amount of revenue you will generate from the money loaned *must* be greater than the total real cost of the loan.

If this is your first time, as an entrepreneur, trying to raise money, keep in mind that you will need detailed projections. You should have a business plan (not an impossible task, really) that describes every facet of your new company, particularly marketing, production, and distribution. A good business plan should include a capital expenditure budget and a projected profit and loss statement. Your banker will take your loan request a lot more seriously if you come prepared with a well-formulated business plan.

The capital expenditure budget lists the cost of your facility (only if you plan on buying it) and equipment (only if you intend to purchase it outright) and any expected physical improvements.

The profit and loss projection shows operation expenses (such as rent, labor, raw materials, packaging materials, and advertising) plus cost of goods sold subtracted from a reasonable estimate of gross sales for a given period. When your prepared profit and loss statement shows a large profit, you should be looking to borrow less or perhaps plan on turning larger portions of revenue back into the business. If it shows even a slight loss, you should plan on borrowing more money over a longer term.

Another thing that you will find helpful is a cash-flow projection (your cash budget). This will forecast the actual cash surplus (extra cash) or deficit (not enough cash) you can expect for each accounting period. Your cash-flow projection shows all the cash you have recorded (payments received, etc.) and your receivables (how much is owed to you). It is a simpler picture of the difference between how much money you've spent and the total amount owed to you in any given month. The expenditures on your cash-flow statement are all-inclusive, containing such items as loan principal, monies for business-related expenses, cash reserved for taxes, etc. A cash-flow statement is helpful in that it can signal cash-shortage problems very early in the game. If you are aware of a deficit (negative cash flow) early enough in a given period of your business growth, you have the opportunity to arrange for additional funding, discuss the possibility of extended credit terms with your suppliers, or cut out some optional expenditures. Suppliers are much more cooperative about working out payment terms if you approach them *before* it becomes a problem.

One more financial statement that you should consider is the balance sheet. Your balance sheet will list what your business owns minus what it owes and its net worth on a given date such as the end of each month, each quarter, or the year.

Very few people (especially those trying to run a new business) like to do extra paperwork. It can be a real pain in the neck. But the time and effort put into this type of bookkeeping will greatly simplify your accounting process (and your life) in the long run.

Please note that it is very important for you to use figures as close to "real" numbers as you can. Being overly optimistic when preparing your original business projections can create problems for you down the road. Consult your local trade associations, trade publications, and suppliers to obtain sound, realistic figures for your industry and product. Dun and Bradstreet also have good numbers available through their *Key Business Ratios* publication. You will have different capital requirements depending on how completely you plan to get involved in the processing operation. Are you going to buy or rent your facility? Will you buy or lease your equipment? What terms will your suppliers offer?

If you do not have enough personal capital to start your business, you will have to decide how you are going to raise the additional funding. The entrepreneur food processor basically has two options.

1. Long-Term Debt. This is your basic business loan. You make arrangements with a bank to lend you the money and you are responsible for paying it back, with interest, within a predetermined period. Long-term debt is costly but it allows you to maintain complete control of your business unless you don't meet the terms of the loan.
2. Equity Financing. In this type of financing, you sell a portion of the rights to your business to an investor. Equity

financing eliminates the worry of loan repayment and interest charges, but you will not be completely in control of your business and you will not receive 100% of your profits.

It is important that you talk with your banker and/or business consultant to determine which type of financing would work best for you. There are all types of packages that can be developed for your particular requirements.

The vast majority of food processors use the type of financing known as "bootstrap" financing. With this kind of financing, you must use your company's internal ability to generate the capital needed to cover your costs. By getting your suppliers to give you generous credit terms (such as net 30 to 60 days), you have some extra time to liquidate inventory produced with these supplies before payment is required. Offer a 2% discount to buyers who pay in full within 10 days of receipt of shipment in order to encourage early payment. By keeping the terms of receivables as short as possible and cutting expenses wherever possible, you may be able to operate your food processing business with minimal outside capital assistance. Bankers and investors seem to look favorably on businesses that practice "tight" business management. If you have a history of maximizing your internal resources, you will usually find it easier to borrow money when funds are required for future expansion. Let's take a more in-depth look at the ways you can maximize your internal resources.

Your customers are the first source of revenue generated by your business. Unfortunately, those of you in the food industry do not have the kind of product or service that can require installment payments or prepayment of goods. You do, however, have a product that has (or should have, if you are going to be successful in this business) a fast turnover time. Most major grocery store chains will not handle a shelf-stable food product that doesn't turn over (placed on the shelf and purchased) every 20–30 days. Because of this kind of turnover, you can expect to be paid for your goods within 30 days. If you have an adequate profit margin and if you would not be cutting into your profits too much, you can "encourage" grocery buyers to pay you within a much shorter period by offering them a discount for early payment. If you can build this discount into your original price and still be able to remain competitive, by all means, do it. If you can get 25% of your customers to pay within 10 days, you will generate that much more working capital and the other 75% of your customers will be paying an additional premium (for holding payment for the full term), which will generate higher revenues. When quoting your original price, it is important to build in a penalty for late payments. Ask around to determine what local standards are for this type of penalty. It's too late to try to charge a penalty after someone is in arrears. All discount and penalty policies must be clearly defined in your original price quotation.

Another good method of internal resource funding lies with your tradespeople or suppliers. They can sometimes be a major source of short-term credit, particularly if you have previously established a solid business relationship with them. It is not unusual for a supplier to extend interest-free credit for 30 days once you have established a satisfactory payment record. The extra 30 days give you the opportunity to liquidate (sell) some of your inventory before the payment is due, eliminating the need for costly bank credit. Keep in mind that it is absolutely imperative that you pay within the terms agreed upon. If you are "unfaithful" to just one of your suppliers, you can count on every other supplier in your region knowing about it and requiring much tighter credit terms from you in the future.

Real estate is another potential form of capital, but keep in mind that too much money invested in real estate can reduce your amount of working capital and threaten your business. You are probably better off renting or leasing your facilities during the early development and growth stages of your food product. However, if you do own your processing facility, you can get additional capital by mortgaging your building or land to banks, commercial finance companies, savings institutions, or insurance companies.

Real estate loans on your commercial property are usually not written for more than 75% of the appraised value of the property. Repayment is usually in monthly installments, amortized over 10 to 30 years. Just as with a regular mortgage, your monthly payments completely pay off the principal and interest by the end of the loan period. You may also have the option of second mortgages, balloon payments, or refinancing. Talk to your banker about these options—he'd be happy to help.

If you spend too much money buying, as opposed to leasing, your processing and packaging equipment, you may find yourself without enough working capital to run your business. This is a very common problem, particularly with new food processors. Sure, that fantastic state-of-the-art equipment would be just the thing for processing your barbecue sauce, but you may have to settle for something a little more labor sensitive until your product starts generating more revenue. If you do decide to buy your equipment, you should consider an equipment loan. Lenders will usually finance 60 to 80% of the equipment's value. The balance represents your down payment on a new purchase or the amount of equity that you retain on your used equipment. The loan is paid in monthly installments (usually calculated on the estimated life of the equipment). Later, if you need extra capital, you can use your already-owned equipment to secure a loan. Banks will typically lend you 70 to 80% of the appraised value of your equipment.

Equipment leasing is another way to avoid typing up all your working capital. Everything you need—from your food processing equipment to your office furniture—can be leased from your bank, commercial finance company, or numerous leasing companies. The lease payments may eventually total more than the original price of the equipment but, by freeing up capital to run your business, the profits generated should more than offset the added cost.

In order for bootstrap financing to work, you must be prepared to keep a very close watch on your business management. Costs must be cut wherever possible, and company resources must be utilized to the maximum advantage. Some things to watch are:

1. Salaries. You must be prepared to pay yourself a lot less than you think you deserve if working capital is short.
2. Company Costs. Be sure you are staying within the same parameters as your competition.
3. Utility Bills. Is there any unnecessary waste of electricity, water, gas, or phone use?
4. Supplies. Are any of your raw materials or packaging materials being wasted?

Keeping a close watch on these types of revenue drains can make or break your business.

Equity Financing

Another type of financing you might want to consider is equity financing. You receive capital for your business operation by giving up a portion of your ownership and profits for a cash investment. Depending on your agreement, your investor may or may not participate in running the business. Many small businesses use equity financing in a limited way. You can often get additional financing from nonprofessional investors such as friends, family or employees. Generally, it is advisable to prepare a written agreement that clearly outlines the terms of the investment. This protects you as well as your non-professional investors and can sometimes save a friendship.

Venture Capitalists

Venture capitalists are a good source of financing for entrepreneurs. They make money available to new, relatively unproven enterprises. Unfortunately, venture capitalist monies are not readily available, particularly for new food processors, because these firms are in the business of investing money to make lots of money. They gamble that an investment in a certain business will return not only their original investment with interest, but with a large profit as well. The food processing industry does not usually generate the kind of profit that venture capitalists find attractive. If you decide to try to attract venture capitalist financing, you will have to have a very strong business plan. Venture capitalists are looking for strong management capabilities, a product with a competitive advantage, and one that fits into a growth-industry classification. Growth industries are those businesses or industries that are growing much faster than the gross national product. (High-tech products often fit this category—food products seldom do!)

Small Business Investment Companies (SBIC)

These are privately owned venture-capital firms eligible for federal loans to be invested in small businesses.

Minority Enterprise Small Business Investment Companies (MESBIC)

These companies are similar to SBIC except that they are restricted to serving only those businesses that are owned at least 51% by socially or economically disadvantaged Americans.

Both SBIC and MESBIC are licensed and regulated by the Small Business Administration (SBA) in Washington. Contact your local SBA for more details and assistance in applying.

Commercial Finance Companies

If your business is new or quickly expanding, you may have some difficulty getting a conventional bank loan. The banks may consider you a risk because your are carrying too high a debt load, or because you have a bad or limited track record, or perhaps because your banker feels it is just too much money to lend you. If you happen to find yourself in this situation, you might want to talk to someone at a local commercial finance company. Finance companies are usually a little more flexible about loaning to small businesses. They are willing to take on a slightly higher risk but with a higher interest rate attached. Finance companies will work with you to package a loan that works best for you.

They are willing to accept collateral in the form of new or used equipment, real estate, or even your account receivables. Commercial finance companies usually do not require as extensive a business plan as venture capitalists or a conventional bank. The most important thing to remember when you are putting together your business financing is to get the best deal possible, but one that you can live with. There are many different resources available to you through state, federal, and local agencies to help you make wise decisions. Shop around before you make any decisions. Proper financing will make or break your business—believe it!

Glossary

Amortize   To pay a debt gradually through scheduled periodic payments; the process of writing off against expenses the cost of an intangible asset over the period of its economic usefulness.

Appreciation   The increase in property value over time.

Balloon payment   The final bulk payment that retires a loan when minimal previous payments have not fully amortized it.

Capital   Net worth of the individual or business; also, the excess of total assets over total liabilities; the funds used to start or *capitalize* a business.

Cash flow   (1) Cash generated from business operation; (2) net income after taxes plus noncash expenses such as depreciation.

Cash (flow) position   The presence or absence of surplus cash for recycling into business operations (sometimes known as "positive" or "negative" cash flow).

Collateral (security)   Personal or real property possessions that the borrower assigns to the lender to help ensure debt payment. If the borrower does not repay the loan, the lender may take ownership of the collateral.

Current assets   Cash or such assets as accounts receivable and inventory that are readily converted to cash during the normal operation of a business cycle, usually within 1 year.

Current liabilities   Debts due within a year, including payments on long-term loans and any anticipated payables such as taxes.

Debentures   The written evidence of a debt, usually issued by a corporation.

Depreciation   The process of writing off against expenses the decrease in value of a fixed asset over its useful life.

Equity (1) The difference between the value of an asset or business and what is owed on it; (2) the money—equity dollars or investment—that purchases ownership.

Fixed assets Permanent business properties such as land, buildings, machinery, and equipment that are *not* resold or converted to cash in normal business operations.

Leverage (1) The extent to which a business is financed by debt; (2) boosting a business's profit potential by injecting debt capital.

Liquidity The degree to which individual or business assets are in cash form or can quickly be converted to cash.

Liquidate To convert noncash assets into cash.

Net working capital The excess of current assets over current liabilities, or the pool of resources readily available for normal business operations.

Prime rate The interest rate set by individual banks for their largest, lowest risk loans—usually, short-term unsecured credit to large creditworthy customers.

, **Term loan** A loan repaid in periodic payments over a period of more than 1 year.

Usury law Ceilings set on loan interest rates by individual states, with exemptions for some competitive commercial lenders. (California's current usury limit exempts state and national banks, savings and loan associations, credit unions, industrial loan companies, pawnbrokers, personal property brokers, agricultural cooperatives, and licensed real estate brokers when the loan is secured by a lien on real property.)

CHAPTER 5

Manufacturing Strategies

It is very important that you develop a workable operations plan, outlining exactly what your manufacturing enterprise is going to entail. Issues such as manufacturing system, site location, inventory management, and quality control standards need to be well thought out and then effectively implemented.

Manufacturing System

When you are structuring the performance criteria necessary for your manufacturing system, there are many things that must be considered.

Investment. What type of capital do you have available to invest in your facility, equipment, production materials, and other inventory?

Unit Cost. What is it going to cost to manufacture this product, including the cost of labor, materials, and overhead? Can you produce the product, add a reasonable profit, and still offer your food product at a competitive price?

Quality. Is your manufacturing process able to produce a high enough percentage of product which meets your quality control standards?

Delivery. Is your system set up to allow for adequate processing time between receipt of order and shipment?

Delivery Reliability. Have you designed enough flexibility into
your system to handle quick growth or seasonal surges
while still meeting delivery schedules?

New Product Capabilities. Have you designed your facility and
manufacturing line in such a way that new products can be
added? You're better off if you design a system that has a lot
of flexibility.

For most companies, all these performance criteria need to
be considered, but it is difficult, if not impossible, to cover all
these variables. Many of these criteria have conflicting objectives. For example, if you have decided that your competitive
product niche is going to be that you are able to deliver your
product more quickly (and thus, fresher) than your competition,
you are going to have to locate your manufacturing facility
closer to your market and/or carry a large inventory of raw
material (for fast processing times) or semifinished product (for
even faster processing times). Holding that type of inventory is
costly. You must measure the importance of one performance
criterion against another. In this case: delivery versus site choice
versus investment. This trading off of the value of one performance criterion against another begins by identifying the
performance measures themselves. This is one of the most
important steps in understanding the manufacturing strategy
for your company.

You will be required to make some very important and
costly decisions about your manufacturing operation. It is
important that you include the following factors in your complete manufacturing strategy:

1. Are you going to buy raw materials or semiprocessed
   goods? Cost is a major factor in this decision, as are
   availability of raw materials and processing capabilities.
   Take, for example, a product like barbecue sauce. If you

are doing your processing in an area where fresh tomatoes are a stable agricultural crop, you would probably
want to plan your major processing times around harvest
"windows." In other words, you'd want to do the majority of your production (at least the tomato base portion of
the process) during the time when tomatoes are readily
available and selling at a good price. You could supplement off-season production with a processed tomato
base, although your profit margins would be affected.

2. What type of equipment should you buy? Processing and
packaging equipment will be one of your major expenses.
Buy good, used equipment whenever possible. Many
companies quickly outgrow their equipment, so there are
usually some excellent deals available. Go to some of the
food processing and packaging equipment trade shows.
There is a major show held in Chicago every year. See
what's available, what's new. It is important that you
look for equipment that is flexible and has several processing capabilities, but don't get caught up in all the
glitzy new technology. When you're just starting up,
you can't afford it. It's like anything else—you'd love a
new Porsche, but a good Ford pick-up truck would be a
wiser choice right now. For more information contact the
following:

Food Processing Machinery and Supplies Association
200 Daingerfield Road
Alexandria, VA 22314
(703) 684-1080

They would be happy to send you resource material and
put you in contact with some of their members who can supply
you with what you need.

Get in touch with some of the excellent trade journals. They
have all kinds of information available to new food processors.
Three good sources are listed as follows:

For prepared foods, contact

The Magazine for Packaged Foods
Gorman Publishing Company
8750 West Bryn Mawr Avenue
Chicago, IL 60631
(312) 693-3200

For food processing, contact

The Magazine of the Food Industry
Putman Publishing Company
301 E. Erie Street
Chicago, IL 60611
(312) 644-2020

And for state-of-the-art technologies, contact

Institute of Food Technologists
221 N. Lasalle Street
Chicago, IL 60601
(312) 782-8424

There are industry-specific journals for almost every facet of the food industry (bakery, dairy, frozen foods, egg, beverage, etc.). Go to your local university library and see what publications they carry. Many of these trade journals are free if you are in the industry.

The following important questions, involving your manufacturing decisions, are answered in this chapter or elsewhere in the book.

1. Will you use an incentive wage or an hourly wage format?
2. Will you build a large inventory on anticipation or structure processing lead time around smaller inventories?
3. Do you want a functional or a product-focused organization?
4. How are you going to handle inventory control?

Site Location

It would seem that one of your relatively easy decisions would be that of where to locate your manufacturing operation and, if you are not investing a great deal of money in your facility, you probably are right. Most new food processors assume that they will manufacture their food product close to where they live. If you are really going to make a serious commitment to this endeavor, there are many other factors which will have to be considered more important than personal convenience. Your main market location and the availability of labor force, raw materials, transportation, and industrial space are all key factors in your site location decision. Proper location of your processing facility is vital to your success. You should begin your location consideration by answering the following questions:

1. Do you need a specialized building or will you be satisfied with an available existing facility?
2. Are there any facilities available that were originally designed for food processing operation? Your banker or a commercial real estate broker who specializes in industrial properties can help you with this.
3. Would it be cheaper to adapt an existing building or to build a new one?

If you decide to build your own facility, there are several things you should keep in mind.

Your Market. Since regional growth is the first market expansion for any small food processor, you need to study your market to see where the largest potential consumer base is located (obviously, this will be close to large metropolitan areas). Since freight and handling is a cost consideration in your pricing structure, the closer you get to your market, the less your cost. Be careful that you don't offset the potential cost savings by locating in a high-priced real estate area.

Your Labor Force. It is important to know that you will have a large enough labor pool to choose from that you will be able to hire good employees. The manufacturing work of food processing doesn't require a PhD, but your employees will be working around expensive, potentially dangerous equipment. One rule of thumb to follow is that the ideal manufacturing facility location is an area that can provide ten persons for consideration for each one to be hired.

Transportation. Have a transportation expert furnish shipping rates and delivery times for your major customers via various modes of transportation. Access to freeways, airports, rail service, and large and deep water transportation should all be considered for your present needs as well as for your future transportation requirements.

Raw Materials. Map out the locations of your sources of raw materials. If they are all located in a relatively central area, you need to consider the advantages of being located adjacent to that area over a more remote facility location.

Is it more important to be closer to raw materials or to your customer? Are these suppliers capable of bringing the raw materials to you rapidly and economically? Can you always be assured of a supply, regardless of season? Does the supply of raw materials from the area seem assured in the foreseeable future? Will the cost of raw materials from the present source change dramatically in the near future?

Suitable Site. Is a suitable site available in the general area in which you have decided to locate? Is needed rail or highway transportation available in the area? Is adequate water and sewer service available?

Local Community Support. Some municipalities aggressively seek new manufacturing facilities. New business creates new jobs, which helps the local economy. If a town or city is eager to have you locate your facility within their community, they may eliminate many of the small problems, such as zoning restrictions, that can arise. Obviously, you should avoid areas that do not want industry or that have a strong no-growth policy. Concentrate on areas that show enthusiasm for you and your business.

The final thing to think about is whether or not you should lease or buy your facility. Some of the questions you should answer before making your decision are listed as follows.

1. Are your manufacturing requirements going to change considerably in the next few years? If they are, you should consider leasing.
2. Do you find yourself in very short supply of capital? Can you use your available money better if it is not tied up in the purchase of a building? What return can you expect from your funds if they are invested elsewhere? If your capital is tight, leasing may be preferable.
3. Can you secure a favorable lease from the owner of the building, perhaps with an option to buy? Because of tax considerations, the property owner may prefer to lease his property rather than sell it. In such a case, he is apt to make the lease price more attractive than the selling price. You should explore this possibility. Talk to your accountant. He can advise you as to how leasing or purchasing might affect your financial picture. If you can buy property at a favorable price and the purchase does not cause a shortage in your working capital, then you might want to seriously consider buying.
4. What would be the potential resale value of the property? Is the building one that will be readily resold? If so, the purchase may be a good one.
5. Are such programs as revenue bonding, tax forgiveness, or other assistance available from your state? Check with your state or local development group to determine what type of help is available (see Appendix B).

You can get local assistance in choosing a site and securing data from a number of sources. Your electric, gas, or telephone utility may have a person who is designated to help companies with their local decisions. Some banks and insurance companies also provide such service. In addition, real estate agents who specialize in commercial and industrial sales, the industrial development department of your local chamber of commerce, as well as the industrial development departments of railway companies can all be of help. State governments usually have departments or agencies which specialize in providing facts for companies considering locating in their areas. There is a lot of assistance out there. Know what you need and what you want, and be prepared to make a smart decision!

Inventory Management

Now that you have your building and your manufacturing strategy, how are you going to control your inventory and the quality of that inventory? These are two very important questions. Your inventory is the most visible and tangible aspect of your food processing operation. Raw materials, finished goods, and goods in process all represent part of your inventory. Your inventory includes all items you have on hand for your manufacturing. These items represent a large portion of your business investment and must be well managed in order to maximize your profit. Your business probably can not afford the types of losses that a poorly managed inventory can cause. Good inventory management involves the following:

1. Maintain a good selection of your product but not too much.
2. Increase inventory turnover but only at a good profit level.
3. Keep processing material stocks as low as possible.
4. Make volume purchases to obtain lower prices but don't overbuy.

Remember, successful inventory management involves simultaneously attempting to balance the costs of inventory with the benefits of inventory. Many small business owners often fail to fully appreciate the true costs of carrying inventory, which include not only direct costs of storage, insurance, and taxes, but also the cost of money tied up in the inventory.

In the beginning stages of your business you will probably need a far less sophisticated system than you think. The number and kinds of records you keep, as well as the type of control system needed, will depend a lot on how many different products you are manufacturing and how much inventory you are going to have on hand. If you are going to use a visual control system you may not need to keep formal records at all. When stock is low, you reorder and/or produce. As you get larger and are carrying more items from various suppliers, you will probably need a more formal inventory system. Records can be kept in a card file. In such a case, regardless of the type of records maintained, the accuracy and discipline of the recorder is critical. It is important to remember that, in many cases, attempts to improve management and reduce costs fail not simply because of insufficient record keeping, but because of inaccurate and carelessly recorded inventory data.

Many small manufacturers, with relatively few items in inventory, use manual inventory control systems. You can use records, inventory tags, and accounting data to capture the information necessary to establish economic order quantities. As your inventory increases, you might want to consider computerizing your system. Small computers capable of handling your inventory system, company accounting, and billing are now available at relatively low prices. More importantly, manufacturers and dealers usually offer free information on the inventory-control software packages available for the various computers.

Whatever type of inventory management system you decide to use, it is important to remember that inventory management involves two separate but closely related elements. The first is knowing what and how much to order, when to order, and what price to pay. The second is making sure that the items, once brought into your inventory, are used properly to produce a profit. The following is an excellent source for some specific inventory management information:

The American Production and Inventory Control Society
2600 Virginia Avenue N.W.
Washington, D.C. 20037

Quality Control Standards

Your quality control standards must be high enough to guarantee that the product you are presenting to the customer is of the highest possible purity, freshness, and quality. If 8–10% of your production run does not pass, your quality control standards are too low. All quality and inspection systems have the following basic elements in common.

Organization. Setting and assigning specific responsibility for each phase of production.

Quality Planning. Writing work instructions with realistic "defect prevention" rules, looking at manufacturing processes for possible quality trouble spots, setting acceptance/rejection standards, controlling disposal or recycling of rejected products, setting up a means of using suppliers' and customers' failure information to improve product quality. Listen to your customers. They are the best group of quality control inspectors available.

Product Specification Control. Making sure each of your operations staff has all the necessary information for properly producing, inspecting, and shipping the product.

Supplier Product Quality Control. Watching purchases to make sure that the people you buy from know and observe your quality requirements.

Measurement and Test Equipment Control. Setting up a system to insure that such equipment is properly and regularly calibrated to establish standards.

Nonconforming Material Control. Spotting defects as early in production as possible and keeping substandard items from reaching customers.

Records and Reports. Setting up a system that tracks all steps of your production, inspection, and shipping cycle to identify existing and potential problem areas.

This may seem like a tremendous amount of extra hassle but, if you take the time to develop a good multifaceted manufacturing plan, you will save yourself lots of problems in the future.

CHAPTER 6

Protecting Yourself and the Consumer

Would you feel comfortable living in a beautiful home, surrounded by priceless possessions, without insuring your estate against fire, flood, or theft? Would you be foolish enough to drive your automobile without insuring yourself against the myriad of possible accidents that can occur while driving? Would you consider yourself a responsible parent if you did not adequately insure your child's health or welfare in the event of your death or disability? Hopefully, you would cover yourself against these potential disasters through various forms of insurance.

There are just as many kinds of insurance available to you as a business person, and many of them are just as important. In the first section of this chapter we will discuss the kinds of insurance you can purchase to protect your business, and in the second section, the types of production precautions you need to take to insure against potential product liabilities. We will also talk briefly about various licenses and permits you will need to stay within the safe parameters of United States law.

Insuring Your Business

Before you begin your manufacturing operation, you should consult with a reputable insurance agent or broker in your area, preferably one who has a background in working with food processors or related industries. He or she will be extremely useful in helping you develop a comprehensive insurance plan which will suit your particular needs.

You will need a fire insurance policy that covers damage to your premises, equipment, and inventory. Fire, smoke, and water can be particularly devastating to certain processed foods. Most packaging cannot stand even slight exposure to any of these elements.

Liability insurance is designed to protect you against financial loss due to any claims of bodily injury or property damage in connection with your production operation. Food processing involves a great deal of chopping, slicing, mashing, and beating at high temperatures. Cuts, bruises, and burns are very common and so, unfortunately, are major injuries. You have to protect your business against normal human accidents, careless or not. Contact your local Occupational Safety and Health Administration (OSHA) office for assistance on this (see Appendix C).

Crime coverage will protect you against losses due to theft, vandalism, or employee dishonesty. This type of insurance is not essential but, with some products and in some geographical regions of the U.S., it may help you sleep at night if you have it.

Automobile insurance covers physical damage and liability for company-owned vehicles or vehicles used for business purposes. It is an absolute must if you have other employees driving your vehicles.

Worker's compensation insurance is mandatory in many states. It protects against liability for employee injuries and loss of pay due to employee accidents incurred while working.

Business interruption insurance is a "peace-of-mind" type of coverage. It would reimburse you for revenue lost during a temporary halt in business due to theft, fire, injury, or illness.

Employee health and life insurance is extremely expensive and often cost prohibitive to a small business. Employees and their dependents are covered in case of illness or death. Programs can be considered that divide the premium cost between employer and employee. This type of insurance is considered an employee benefit and may be a deciding factor for potential employees, particularly management.

Product liability insurance protects the business from claims against a defective product. It is very important for a food manufacturer, particularly with products that have the potential for being hazardous to consumer health if there should be a processing problem. More and more major grocery outlets are requiring some kind of manufacturer's guarantee on this kind of liability.

Because of the various problems and potential health hazards involved in food production, the U.S. Government has established some pretty strict guidelines that you will have to follow. It is an unfortunate fact that most small food product manufacturers are not aware of the various laws regarding their products and the manufacturing of their products. This lack of knowledge has caused many small business persons to find themselves in legal difficulty.

U.S. consumers are protected from potential health hazards relating to food, drugs, and cosmetics by the U.S. Department of Health and Human Services, the Public Health Service, and the Food and Drug Administration (FDA). It is the responsibility of the FDA to enforce both laws enacted by the U.S. Congress and regulations developed by the Agency to protect the consumer's health, safety, and pocketbook. It is the responsibility of any person producing food products commercially to know and comply with these regulations.

The Federal Food, Drug, and Cosmetic Act (21 USC 301–392) is the basic food and drug law of the United States. It relates to imported food products as well as all food processed in the U.S. that travels across state lines. With numerous amendments, it is the most extensive law of its kind in the world. Many other countries have modeled their regulations after ours. Food products that are manufactured and stay within the borders of one state are generally governed only by the laws and regulations of that state, but the federal law may sometimes apply even to these products. Many of the states in the U.S. have laws similar to the federal law, and some have provisions to automatically add any new federal requirements. The law is intended to assure the consumer that foods are pure and wholesome, safe to eat, and produced under strict sanitary conditions.

Each state has its own regulations regarding food processing. A state agency (usually the Health Department or a division of the state's Department of Agriculture) will handle inspections of all facilities where food is prepared for human consumption. You are usually not given any notice that you will be inspected; the inspector just shows up at your facility unannounced.

If he or she finds any violations, you are given a specified amount of time to rectify the situation. If you have an excessive number of violations, or if you do not "clean up" the problem areas, the inspector has complete authority to shut down your operation until such time as you do pass the inspection.

Included here is a sample of a typical inspection form. Each state's form is different but by and large they all contain the same inspection points (see Figure 6.1).

Another law, the Fair Packaging and Labeling Act (15 USC 1451–1461), affects the contents and placement of information required on packaging. This law strictly requires that labeling and packaging be truthful, informative, and not deceptive. To avoid problems, all food processors should clear their product and packaging with their local FDA office (a list of these offices appears at the end of this chapter) before the product reaches the shelf.

An excellent example of the government's swift (and effective) action is the recent Beech-Nut baby food scandal.[1] In this particular case the former President/CEO and former Vice President of Manufacturing were indicted in 1986 by the U.S. Government, under FDA directives, for selling mislabeled and adulterated apple juice for infants. The product was labeled 100% natural juice when, in actuality, it was a concentrate base, heavily laced with chemical preservative. The men were sentenced in 1988 to a year and a day in prison and fined $100,000 each. Aside from the horrible mess both of these gentlemen

[1]Source: FDA Consumer, June 1988; Business Week, February, 1988.

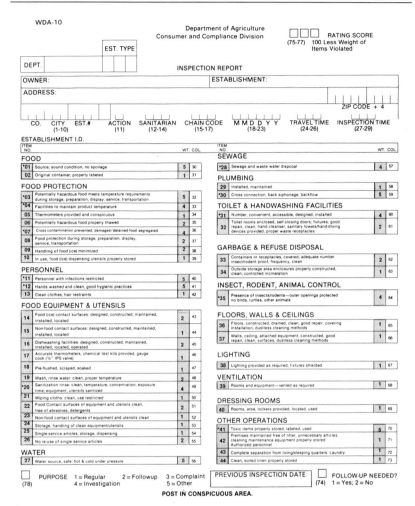

Figure 6.1   Sample of a typical inspection form.

made of their lives, the Beech-Nut Company is experiencing a severe sales slump in a baby food market that is growing 9–10% a year.

As with most other laws, you will find that the various regulations and explanations of the Food and Drug Act are available in a book the size of the Los Angeles phone book. It is very important that you contact your regional representative of the

FDA. The staff of the FDA are very knowledgeable and they will help you identify exactly which regulations your particular product needs to comply with.Give them a call—after all, they work for you. Your taxes pay their salaries.

Briefly summarized, here are some of the more important portions of the law that you will need to know and comply with.

First, let's touch upon the rules that apply to everyone involved in the manufacturing, distributing, or importing of food. The Federal Food, Drug, and Cosmetic Act prohibits distribution in the U.S. of food articles that are adulterated or misbranded. The term "adulterated" includes products that are defective, unsafe, filthy, or produced under unsanitary conditions. "Misbranded" includes statements, designs, or pictures in labeling that are false or misleading and failure to provide required information in labeling. For example, a frozen entree producer cannot use a picture of a beautiful prime rib being sliced off the beef when his dinner product actually contains "restructured beef." Another good example of mislabeling can occur when products claiming to be oven roasted, hickory smoked, or barbecued are actually flavor enhanced with chemicals. The FDA monitors processing claims such as these very closely.Detailed definitions of adulteration and misbranding are in the law itself and hundreds of court decisions have interpreted them. You don't want to get hit with noncompliance of any of these.

Another very important part of the law prohibits the distribution of any article required to be approved by the FDA if such approval has not been given. It also prohibits the food manufacturer from refusing to provide required reports or from refusing unscheduled inspections of regulated facilities. This brings us to an important bit of information. Within the U.S., compliance with the Food, Drug, and Cosmetic Act is secured through periodic inspection of facilities and products, analysis of samples, educational activities, and legal proceedings. When violations of the act are discovered, there are many regulatory procedures available. All of them spell TROUBLE and/or major inconvenience for the small business person. Adulterated or misbranded products may be voluntarily destroyed or recalled from the market by the shipper, or they may be seized by U.S. Marshals on orders obtained by the FDA from the federal district courts. Persons or firms responsible for violations may be prosecuted in federal court and, if found guilty, may be fined and/or imprisoned.

When FDA investigators observe unsanitary conditions or practices which may result in violations, they leave a written report of their observations with management. Manufacturers must bring their operations into compliance by correcting these conditions or practices promptly. In the event you do not comply, the FDA has the right to recall the product. Product recall has become an effective means of consumer protection under the law. It is also an effective way for the food manufacturer to avoid a court appearance and possible consequences. Voluntary recall on the part of the manufacturer is generally the fastest and most effective way to protect the public. It is not uncommon to hear of a national-level recall of a product when only one contaminated package has been identified. (Remember how Chilean fruit imports came to a dramatic halt in March of 1989 when only two grapes were found to contain a relatively harmless amount of cyanide?) In 1987, a major tuna packer recalled a full production run (several thousand cans) because a consumer had become seriously ill from consuming the product. The cost of this kind of recall can be devastating, but the potential liability and bad press can be worse. Incidentally, if the tuna packer had not reacted so quickly and without such a high level of responsibility, the FDA had the right to pull all his product off the shelf. A recall may be requested by the manufacturer, the shipper, or the FDA. While cooperation in a recall may make court proceedings unnecessary in removing the product from the market, it does not release a firm from liability for the violation.

Another method available to the FDA is the right to seizure of your product. Seizure is a civil court action to remove goods from the channels of commerce. After seizure, the goods may not be altered, used, or moved. The food manufacturer is responsible for all storage charges. This kind of action can easily bankrupt the small business person, so it should be avoided at the outset. The owner or claimant of the seized merchandise is usually given about 30 days by the court to decide on the course of action. He may do nothing, in which case the goods will be disposed of by the court. He may decide to contest the government's charges by filing a claim and answering the charges, at which time the case will be scheduled for trial. Keep in mind that the court system is notoriously slow, and this could take months, if not years. Meanwhile, you are paying storage fees and your product's shelf life is rapidly expiring. The claimant may also decide to consent to condemnation of the goods while requesting permission from the court to bring the goods into compliance with the law. In this case, the owner is required to provide a bond (deposit of money) to ensure that the orders of the court will be carried out and must pay for the FDA supervision of any compliance procedures.

The federal government has created very powerful assurances to encourage compliance by food manufacturers with the Food, Drug, and Cosmetic Act. It makes sense for any food manufacturer, big or small, to know and respect these rules in advance.

The following section contains a summary of the Federal Food, Drug, and Cosmetic Act's food-related regulations. (U.S. Department of Health and Human Services, Food and Drug Administration. U.S. Government Printing Office, Washington, D.C.)

Food-Related Regulations

Section 201(f) of the Federal Food, Drug, and Cosmetic Act defines "food" as follows: (1) articles used for food or drink for man or other animals; (2) chewing gum; and (3) articles used for components of any such article.

Principal Requirements of Food Law

Below is a synopsis of the principal requirements of the Act relating to foods, in nonlegal language. The numbers in parentheses or braces are the pertinent sections of the statute itself, or sections in the Code of Federal Regulations (CFR).

Health Safeguards

A food is illegal (adulterated) if it bears or contains an added poisonous or deleterious (harmful) substance which *may* render it injurious to health [402(a)(1)].

A food is illegal if it bears or contains a naturally occurring poisonous or deleterious substance which *ordinarily* renders it injurious to health [402(a)(1)].

Food additives [201(s)] must be determined to be safe by the FDA before they may be used in a food or become a part of a food as a result of processing, packaging, transporting, or holding the food (409).

Raw agricultural products are illegal if they contain residues of pesticides not authorized by, or in excess of, tolerances established by regulations of the Environmental Protection Agency (408).

A food is illegal if it is prepared, packed, or held under insanitary conditions whereby it *may* have been rendered injurious to health [402(a)(4)].

Food containers must be free from any poisonous or deleterious substance which may cause the contents to be injurious to health [402(a)(6)]. Some packaging materials, for example, plastic or vinyl containers, may be "food additives" subject to regulations (409).

Only those colors found safe by the Food and Drug Administration may be added to food (706). A food is illegal if it bears or contains an unsafe color(s) [402(c)]. Unless exempt by regulation, colors for use in food must be from batches tested and certified by the Food and Drug Administration [706(c)].

A food is illegal if any part of it is filthy, putrid, or decomposed [402(a)(3)].

A food is illegal if it is prepared, packed, or held under unsanitary conditions whereby it may have become contaminated with filth [402(a)(4)].

A food is illegal if it is the product of a diseased animal or one that has died otherwise than by slaughter [402(a)(5)].

Economic Safeguards

Damage or inferiority in food must not be concealed in any manner [402(b)(3)]. For example, artificial coloring or flavoring may not be added to a food to make it appear a better value than it is, as in the case of yellow coloring used to make a food appear to contain more eggs than it actually contains.

Food labels or labeling (circulars, etc.) must not be false or misleading in any particular [403(a)]. Labeling is misleading not only if it contains false or misleading statements but also if it fails to reveal material facts [201(n)].

A food must not be sold under the name of another food [403(b)], for example, canned bonito labeled as tunafish.

A substance recognized as being a valuable constituent of a food must not be omitted or abstracted in whole or in part, nor may any substance be substituted for the food in whole or in part [402(b)(1) and (2)], for example, an article labeled "milk" or "whole milk" from which part of the butterfat has been skimmed.

Food containers must be so made, formed, or filled as to be misleading [403(d)], for example, a closed package filled to less than its capacity. A food for which a standard of fill of container has been prescribed (402) must comply with the fill requirements, and if the fill falls below that specified its label must bear a statement that it falls below such standard [403(h)(2)].

Required Label Statements

The law states that required label information must be conspicuously displayed and in terms that the ordinary consumer is likely to read and understand under ordinary conditions of purchase and use [403(f)].

Details concerning type sizes, location, etc., of required label information are contained in FDA Regulations (21 CFR 101), which cover the requirements of both the Federal Food, Drug, and Cosmetic Act and the Fair Packaging and Labeling Act. Food labeling requirements of the regulations are summarized as follows.

If the label of a food bears representations in a foreign language, the label must bear all of the required statements in the foreign language as well as in English. (Note: The Tariff Act of 1930 requires all imported articles to be marked with the English name of the country of origin.)

If the food is packaged, the following statements must appear on the label in the English language:

1. The name, street address, city, state and zip code of the manufacturer, the packer, or the distributor. The street address may be omitted by a firm listed in a current city or telephone directory. A firm whose address is outside the United States may omit the zip code. If the food is not manufactured by the person or company whose name appears on the label, the name must be qualified by "Manufactured for," "Distributed by," or similar expression.

2. An accurate statement of the net amount of food in the package. The required units of measure are the avoirdupois pound and the U.S. gallon, but metric system measurements may also be used, if desired, in addition to the required declaration in "English" units. The quantity of contents declaration must appear on the principal display panel of the label in lines generally parallel to the base of the package when displayed for sale. If the area of the principal display panel of the package is larger than 5 square inches, the quantity of contents must appear within the lower 30% of the label. The declaration must be in a type size based upon the area of the principal display panel of the package (as listed in 21 CFR 101.105) and must be separated from the other information.

The net weight on packages containing 1 pound (avoirdupois) or more and less than 4 pounds must be declared first in total avoirdupois ounces followed by a second statement in parentheses ( ) in terms of pounds and ounces or pounds and common or decimal fractions of the pound [For example, Net Wt. 24 ounces (1½ pounds) or Net Wt. 24 oz. (1.5 lb.).] The contents of packages containing less than 1 pound must be expressed as total ounces.

Drained weight rather than net weight is required on some products packed in a liquid that is not consumed as food, such as olives in brine.

Net volume of liquid products in packages containing 1 pint or more and less than 1 U.S. gallon must be declared first in total fluid ounces followed by a second statement in parentheses in terms of quarts, pints, and fluid ounces or fractions of the pint or quart. [For example, 40 fluid ounces (1.25 quarts) or 40 fluid ounces (1¼ quarts).] Volume of packages containing less than 1 pint must be declared in fluid ounces.

Packages 4 pounds or larger or 1 gallon or larger need not have their contents expressed in terms of total ounces; however, for such packages the contents must be stated in the largest unit of weight or measure, with any remainder in ounces or common or decimal fractions of the pound; or in the case of gallons, the remainder in quarts, pints, and fluid ounces, or decimal fractions of the gallon. If the label of any food package also represents the contents in terms of the number of servings, the size of each serving must be indicated.

3. The common or usual name of a food. This must appear on the principal display panel, in bold type and in lines generally parallel to the base of the package as it is displayed. The form of the product must also be included—"sliced," "whole," or "chopped" (or other style)—unless shown by a picture or unless the product is visible through the container. If there is a standard for the food, the complete name designated in the standard must be used, limitations must be labeled as such [403(e) and 21 CFR 101.3].

4. The ingredients in a food. These must be listed by their common names in order of their predominance by weight unless the food is standardized, in which case the label must include only those ingredients which the standard makes optional. Most ingredients in standardized foods are "optional" and therefore must be listed on the label. The word *ingredients* does not refer to the chemical composition, but means the individual food components of a mixed food. If a certain ingredient is the characterizing one in a food (e.g., shrimp in shrimp cocktail) the percentage of that ingredient may be required as part of the name of the food.

Food additives and colors are required to be listed as ingredients, but the law exempts butter, cheese, and ice cream from having to show the use of color. Spices, flavors, and colors may be listed as such without naming the specific materials, but any artificial colors or flavors must be identified as such, and certain coal-tar colors must be named specifically [403(i) and 430(k)].

Foods for Special Dietary Uses

Section 403(j) of the Food, Drug, and Cosmetic Act classes a food as misbranded "If it purports to be or is represented for special dietary uses, unless its label bears such information concerning its vitamin, mineral, and other dietary properties as the Secretary determines to be, and by regulations prescribes as, necessary in order fully to inform purchasers as to its value for such uses."

Section 411(c)(3) of the Act defines "special dietary use" as a particular use for which a food purports or is represented to be used, including but not limited to the following:

1. Supplying a special dietary need that exists by reason of a physical, physiological, pathological, or other condition, including but not limited to the conditions of disease, convalescence, pregnancy, lactation, infancy, allergic

hypersensitivity to food, underweight, or the need to control the intake of sodium.

2. Supplying a vitamin, mineral, or other ingredient for use by humans to supplement the diet by increasing the total dietary intake.

3. Supplying a special dietary need by reason of being a food for use as the sole item of the diet.

Regulations under this section of the Act (21 CFR 105) prescribe appropriate information and statements which must be given on the labels of foods in this class.

Importers and foreign shippers should consult the detailed regulations under sections 403(j) and 411 and 412 before importing foods represented by labeling or otherwise as special dietary foods.

When special dietary foods are labeled with claims of disease prevention, treatment, mitigation, cure, or diagnosis, they must comply with the drug provisions of the Act.

Infant Foods

The Infant Formula Act of 1980 (21 USC 412) amended the Federal Food, Drug, and Cosmetic Act to establish nutrient requirements for infant formulas and to give FDA authority to establish requirements for quality control, record keeping, reporting, and recall procedures. The Act also extends the FDA's factory inspection authority to permit access to manufacturers' records and test results necessary to determine compliance.

The Act specifies that an infant formula is adulterated (1) if it fails to provide nutrients as required; (2) if it fails to meet the nutrient quality factors required by regulation; or (3) if the processing is not in compliance with appropriate quality control procedures or record retention requirements as prescribed by regulation. Formulas for infants with inborn errors of metabolism or other unusual medical or dietary problems are exempted.

Under authority of the Act, the FDA has promulgated regulations which specify the quality control and recall procedures for infant formulas. Current labeling regulations (21 CFR 105.65) specify the kind of label information that must be present on these foods in addition to the mandatory label information required on all packaged foods. These regulations, however, predate the Infant Formula Act and are being revised. In addition, the FDA has proposed regulations on foods for infants with special medical or dietary needs. Inquiries should be directed to the Food and Drug Administration, Division of Regulatory Guidance (HFF-314), 200 C Street, S.W., Washington, D.C. 20204.

Nutrition Labeling

Whenever a vitamin, mineral, or protein is added to a food product (as in fortification or enrichment) or when the label, labeling, or advertising claims some nutritional value (such as "rich in vitamin C"), the label must have a panel of information about the nutritional quality of that food. The kind of information that must be provided is described in the *Code of Federal Regulations* (21 CFR 101.9). As a minimum, the required labeling calls for listing the size of a serving, the number of servings in the container, the amount of calories, protein, carbohydrate, and fat per serving, and the percentages per serving of the "U.S. Recommended Daily Allowances" (U.S. RDAs) of protein and seven vitamins and minerals. Other nutrients recognized as essential in the human diet may be listed if they contribute at least 2% of the U.S. RDA. The regulations also specify the location and conspicuousness of the required information.

For the benefit of persons who are on a fat-modified diet, the information may include declarations of cholesterol content and the content of saturated and polyunsaturated fatty acids (21 CFR 101.25).

The U.S. RDAs are derived from dietary standards established by the National Academy of Sciences to serve as goals for good nutrition.

Sodium labeling regulations, published in the *Federal Register* April 18, 1984, provide for information on food labels to enable consumers to avoid excessive salt and sodium in their diets. Studies have shown that high blood pressure, a leading cause of heart attacks and stroke, may be associated with excessive sodium intake in susceptible individuals. The rules amend the FDA's food labeling regulations to require that nutrition labeling include the amount of sodium in milligrams per serving. Sodium information may also be voluntarily provided in the absence of nutrition labeling. Quantitative standards and label terminology for sodium declarations are established as follows:

"Sodium free"—less than 5 mg per serving
"Very low sodium"—35 mg or less per serving
"Low Sodium"—140 mg or less per serving
"Reduced sodium"—processed to reduce the usual level of sodium by 75%.
"Unsalted"—processed without salt when the food normally is processed with salt.

Voluntary compliance began when the rules were published, to become mandatory July 1, 1985 for all affected products marketed after this date. Further information is obtainable from the Food and Drug Administration (HFF-204) 200 C Street, S.W., Washington, D.C. 20204.

Sanitation Requirements

One of the basic purposes of the Food, Drug, and Cosmetic Act is protection of the public from products that may be deleterious, that are unclean or decomposed, or that have been exposed to unsanitary conditions that may contaminate the product with filth or may render it injurious to health.

Sanitation provisions of the Food, Drug, and Cosmetic Act go further than to prohibit trade in products that are carriers of disease. The law also requires that foods be produced in sanitary facilities. It prohibits distribution of foods which may contain repulsive or offensive matter considered as filth regardless of whether such objectionable substances can be detected in the laboratory. Filth includes contaminants such as rat, mouse, and other animal hairs and excreta, whole insects, insect parts and excreta, parasitic worms, pollution from the excrement of man and animals, as well as other extraneous materials which, because of their repulsiveness, would not knowingly be eaten or used. The presence of such filth renders foods adulterated, whether or not harm to health can be shown.

The law thus requires that food be protected from contamination at all stages of production. Such protection includes extermination and exclusion of rodents, inspection and sorting of raw materials to eliminate the insect-infested and decomposed portions, quick handling and proper storage to prevent insect development or contamination, the use of clean equipment, control of possible sources of sewage pollution, and supervision of personnel who prepare foods so that acts of misconduct may not defile the products they handle.

Foods that are free from contamination when they are shipped sometimes become contaminated en route and must be detained or seized. This emphasizes the importance of insisting on proper storage conditions in vessels, railroad cars, or other conveyances. While the shipper may be blameless, the law requires action against illegal merchandise no matter where it may have become illegal. All shippers should pack their products so as to protect them against spoilage or contamination en route, and should urge carriers to protect the merchandise by maintaining sanitary conditions and segregating food from other cargo which might contaminate it. For example, vessels transporting foods may also carry ore concentrates and poisonous insecticides. Improper cargo handling or disasters at sea have resulted in shipments becoming seriously contaminated, with detentions required.

Where import shipments become contaminated after customs entry and landing (for example, in truck accidents, fires, barge sinkings, etc.), legal actions are not taken under the import provisions of the law, but by seizure proceedings in a federal district court, as with domestic interstate shipments (304).

Fumigation of commodities already infested with insects will not result in a legal product since dead insects or evidence of past insect activity are objectionable. Fumigation may be employed where necessary to *prevent* infestation, but care is required to prevent buildup of nonpermitted chemical residues from fumigation.

Current Good Manufacturing Practice Regulations

To explain what is needed to maintain sanitary conditions in food establishments, the FDA has published a set of Current Good Manufacturing Practice Regulations. These tell what kinds of buildings, facilities, equipment, and maintenance are needed, and the errors to avoid, to ensure sanitation. They also deal with such matters as building design and construction, lighting, ventilation, toilet and washing facilities, cleaning of equipment, materials handling, and vermin control. Food firms which do not have copies of these regulations are urged to request them by writing to the Food and Drug Administration.

Many food materials are intended for further processing and manufacture into finished foods. Such processing in no way relieves the raw materials from the requirements of cleanliness and freedom from deleterious impurities.

Tolerances for Filth

Many inquiries are received by the Food and Drug Administration as to permitted variations from absolute cleanliness or soundness in foods. The Act does not explicitly provide for "tolerances" for filth or decomposition in foods. It states that a food is adulterated if it consists *in whole or in part* of a filthy, putrid, or decomposed substance.

This does not mean that a food must be condemned because of the presence of foreign matter in amounts below the irreducible minimum after all possible precautions have been taken. The FDA recognizes that it is not possible to grow, harvest, and process crops that are totally free of natural defects. The alternative—to increase the use of chemicals to control insects, rodents, and other sources of contamination—is not acceptable because of the potential health hazards from chemical residues. To resolve the problem the FDA has published a list of "defect action levels," stating the amounts of contamination which will subject the food to enforcement action. Copies may be obtained by request to the nearest FDA office.

The *Food Defect Action Levels* are established at levels that pose no hazard to health and may be changed from time to time. Any products which might be harmful to consumers are subject to regulatory action, whether or not they exceed the "defect" levels. In addition, manufacturing processes that do not conform to the FDA's Current Good Manufacturing Practice Regulations will result in regulatory action by the FDA whether or not the product exceeds the defect action level. The levels are not averages—actually the average levels are much lower, and the FDA continues to lower the action levels as industry performance improves. The mixing of food to dilute contamination is prohibited and renders the product illegal regardless of any defect level in the final product.

Food Additives

"Food additives" are substances which may by their intended uses become components of food, either directly or indirectly, or which may otherwise affect the characteristics of the food. The term specifically includes any substance intended for use in producing, manufacturing, packing, processing, preparing, treating, packaging, transporting, or holding the food, and any source of radiation intended for any such use (409).

But the law excludes the following from the definition of a "food additive":

1. Substances generally recognized as safe by qualified experts;
2. Substances used in accordance with a previous approval ("prior sanction") under the Federal Food, Drug, and

Cosmetic Act, the Poultry Products Inspection Act (21 USC 451), or the Meat Inspection Act;
3. Pesticide chemicals in or on raw agricultural products;
4. A color additive;
5. A new animal drug [but these (3, 4 and 5) are subject to similar safety requirements of other sections of the law].

Manufacturers or importers not certain whether the chemicals or other ingredients used in their foods are subject to the safety clearance requirements of the Food Additives Amendment may seek an opinion from the Food and Drug Administration. If premarket approval is required, this may mean that studies, including animal feeding tests, will have to be carried out in accordance with recognized scientific procedures and the result submitted to the Food and Drug Administration for evaluation. General principles for evaluating the safety of food additives are published in 21 CFR 170.20. Detailed instructions for preparing a food additive petition are in 21 CFR 171. The "Delaney Clause" in the law [409(c)(3)] provides that no food additive may be found safe if it produces cancer when ingested by man or animals or if it is shown by other appropriate tests to be a cancer-producing agent, except that such ingredient may be used in animal feeds if it causes no harm to the animal and provided there are no residues of the ingredient in the meat or other edible products reaching the consumer. This later provision is primarily applicable to veterinary drugs added to animal feed.

If the Food and Drug Administration concludes from the evidence submitted to it that the additive will be safe, a regulation permitting its use will be issued. This regulation may specify the amount of the substance which may be present in or on the foods, the foods in which it is permitted, the manner of use, and any special labeling required.

A substance cleared under the Food Additive Regulations is still subject to all general requirements of the Food, Drug, and Cosmetic Act.

The Saccharin Study and Labeling Act, passed November 23, 1977, prohibited for 18 months any new regulations restricting or banning the sale of saccharin or products containing it. Congress has extended the legislation three times, most recently through 1985. It requires further scientific evaluation of the carcinogenic potential of saccharin, and a label warning: "Use of this product may be hazardous to your health. This product contains saccharin, which has been determined to cause cancer in laboratory animals."

Artificially sweetened products are required to be labeled as Special Dietary Foods (21 CFR 105.66). The foods permitted to contain such sweeteners, and the amounts, are specified in the Food Additive Regulations (21 CFR 180.37).

Housewares

Anyone manufacturing food-contact articles for use in the home or in food-service establishments should make sure that nothing from the articles imparts flavor, color, odor, toxicity, or other undesirable characteristics to food, thereby rendering the food adulterated.

While food packaging materials are subject to regulation as "food additives," ordinary housewares are not. Such housewares include dishes, flatware, beverage glasses, mugs, cooking utensils, cutlery, and electrical appliances. This means that manufacturers do not have to submit data to the FDA showing that the materials used are safe. They also are not required to preclear their housewares with the FDA. But housewares are not exempt from the general safety provisions of the Federal Food, Drug, and Cosmetic Act. Regulatory actions have been taken against cookware and ceramic dinnerware containing lead or cadmium.

Food Standards

Food standards are a necessity to both consumers and the food industry. They maintain the nutritional values and the general quality of a large part of the national food supply. Without standards, different foods would have the same names and the same foods different names, both situations confusing and misleading consumers and creating unfair competition.

Section 401 of the Federal Food, Drug, and Cosmetic act requires that whenever such action will promote honesty and fair dealing in the interest of consumers, regulations shall be promulgated fixing and establishing for any food, under its common or usual name so far as practicable, a reasonable definition and standard of identity, a reasonable standard of quality, and/or reasonable standards of fill of container. However, no definition and standard of identity or standard of quality may be established for fresh or dried fruits, fresh or dried vegetables, or butter, except that definitions and standards of identity may be established for avocados, cantaloupes, citrus fruits, and melons.

Standards of identity define what a given food product is, its name and the ingredients which must be used, or may be used, and which ones must be declared on the label. *Standards of quality* are minimum standards only and establish specifications for quality requirements. *Fill of container* standards define how full the container must be and how this is measured. FDA standards are based on the assumption that the food is properly prepared from clean, sound materials. Standards do not usually relate to such factors as deleterious impurities, filth, and decomposition. There are exceptions. For example, the standards for whole egg and yolk products and for egg white products require these products to be pasteurized or otherwise treated to destroy all viable *Salmonella* microorganisms. Some standards for foods set nutritional requirements such as those for enriched bread, or nonfat dry milk with added vitamins A and D, etc. A food which is represented or purports to be a food for which a standard of identity has been promulgated must comply with the specifications of the standard in every respect.

A food that imitates another food is misbranded unless its label bears in type of uniform size and prominence the word *imitation* and immediately thereafter the name of the food imitated [403(c)]. Under the law a food is an *imitation food* if it is a substitute for and resembles another food but is nutritionally inferior to that food. But if the food is not nutritionally inferior to the food it imitates, it is permitted to be labeled descriptively according to the regulations in 21 CFR 101.3(e) and need not bear the term "imitation."

Standards of quality established under the Food, Drug, and Cosmetic Act must not be confused with *standards for grades* that are published by the U.S. department of Agriculture for meat and other agricultural products and the U.S. Department of the Interior for fishery products. A standard of quality under the Food, Drug, and Cosmetic Act is a minimum standard only. If a food for which a standard of quality or fill of container has been promulgated falls below such standard, it must bear in a prescribed size and style of type label statements showing it to be substandard in quality, or in fill of container; for example, ""Below Standard in Quality, Good Food—Not High Grade."

The U.S. Department of Agriculture grades which have been established are usually designated "Grade A" or "Fancy," "Grade B" or "Choice," or "Grade C" or "Standard." The U.S. Department of the Interior grades for fishery products are usually designated "Grade A," "Grade B," or "Grade C." These grade designations are not required by the Food, Drug, and Cosmetic Act to be stated on the labels, but if they are stated, the product must comply with the specifications for the declared grade.

Fill of container standards established for certain foods designate the quantity in terms of the solid or liquid components, or both. The existing fill-of-container standards for canned fruits and vegetables may be grouped as follows: (1) those that require the maximum practicable quantity of the solid food that can be sealed in the container and processed by heat without crushing or breaking such component (limited to canned peaches, pears, apricots, and cherries); (2) those requiring a minimum quantity of the solid food in the container after processing. The quantity is commonly expressed either as a minimum drained weight for a given container size or as a percentage of the water capacity of the container; (3) those requiring that the food, including both solid and liquid packing medium, shall occupy not less than 90% of the total capacity of the container; (4) those requiring both a minimum drained weight and the 90% minimum fill; and (5) those requiring a minimum volume of the solid component irrespective of the quantity of liquid (canned green peas and canned field peas). Fill-of-container standards specifying minimum net weight or minimum drained weight have been promulgated for certain fish products. The specific requirements of these standards are discussed in other sections of this manual.

FDA food standards govern both labeling and composition and should be consulted for detailed specifications. The standards are published in the annual editions of the *Code of Federal Regulations* (Title 21, Parts 103-169).

International Food Standards (the Codex Alimentarius) have been developed by committees of the World Health Organization and the Foreign Agriculture Organization of the United Nations, of which the United States is a member. The U.S. Government may adopt Codex standards in whole or in part, in accordance with the procedures outlined in the preceding paragraph.

The following sections provide pertinent information on requirements for specific groups of foods.

Canned Foods

Low-Acid Canned Foods and Acidified Foods Regulations

Special regulations apply to the manufacture of heat-processed low-acid canned foods and acidified foods (21 CFR 108, 113, and 114).

The purpose of these regulations is to ensure safety from harmful bacteria or their toxins, especially the deadly *Clostridium botulinum*. This can only be accomplished by adequate processing, controls, and appropriate processing methods, such as cooking the food at the proper temperatures for sufficient times, adequately acidifying the food, or controlling water activity.

Low-acid canned foods are heat-processed foods other than alcoholic beverages that have an acidity greater than pH 4.6 and a water activity (a_w) greater than 0.85 and which are packaged in hermetically sealed containers. "Water activity" is a measure of the water available for microbial growth. A hermetically sealed container is any package, regardless of its composition (i.e, metal, glass, plastic, polyethylene-lined cardboard, etc.), that is capable of maintaining the commercial sterility of its contents after processing. Acidified foods are low-acid foods to which acid(s) or acid food(s) are added to reduce the pH to 4.6 or below (increase the acidity) and with a water activity greater than 0.85. Pimientos, artichokes, some puddings, and some sauces are examples of acidified foods. Questions about product status can be referred to the FDA at the address given below.

The regulations, first adopted in 1973 and revised in 1979, are based on proposals made by the canning industry following FDA investigations of deaths and illness from botulism associated with lax practices in low-acid canned food and acidified food processing.

All commercial processors of low-acid canned foods and acidified foods are required to register their establishments and file processing information for all products with the Food and Drug Administration, using appropriate forms. Registration and process filing is required for both U.S. establishments and those in other countries which export such foods to the United States (21 CFR 108.25 and 108.35).

Registration and processing forms and information are obtainable on request from: Food and Drug Administration, LACF Registration Coordinator (HFF-233), 200 C Street, S.W., Washington, D.C. 20204.

In addition to the registration and process filing requirements, processors must comply with other mandatory provisions of 21 CFR 108 as well as Parts 113 and 114. The mandatory provisions are always preceded by the word *shall*.

Canned Fruits and Fruit Juices

Standards of identity, quality, and fill of container have been promulgated for a number of canned fruits and fruit juices. The specific standards should be consulted by anyone intending to ship canned fruit to the United States.

Labels on canned fruits and fruit juices which meet the minimum quality standards and canned fruits and fruit juices for which no standards of quality have been promulgated need not make reference to quality, but if they do, the product must correspond to the usual understanding of the labeled grade. Particular care must be taken to use the terms "Fancy" or "Grade A" only on those products meeting the specifications established for such grades by the U.S. Department of Agriculture.

Fill-of-Container Standards—Fruits and Juices

Fill-of-container standards have been promulgated for a number of canned fruits and fruit juices, but in packing any other canned fruit the container must be well filled with the fruit and with only enough packing medium added to fill the interstices: otherwise the container may be deceptive and prohibited by the Act. In judging the finished product, due allowance is made for natural shrinkage in processing.

The standards of fill for *canned peaches, pears, apricots, and cherries* require that the fill of the solid food component be the maximum practicable quantity that can be sealed in the container and processed by heat without crushing or breaking such component.

Standards for *canned fruit cocktail, grapefruit, and plums* specify minimum drained weights for the solid food component, expressed as a percentage of the water capacity of the container. These drained weight requirements are as follows: fruit cocktail, 65%; grapefruit, 50%; whole plums, 50%; and plum halves, 55%. An additional 90% fill requirement based on the total capacity of the container for the solid food and the liquid packing medium have been established for plums. This 90% fill requirement also applies to applesauce in metal containers (85% fill for applesauce in glass), crushed pineapple, and pineapple juice.

Minimum drained weight requirements for canned pineapple provide that "crushed pineapple" may be labeled as "heavy pack" or "solid pack." The standard of quality requires a minimum drained weight for crushed pineapple of 63% of the net weight.

All fruit used for canning or juice should be mature and sound, that is, free from insect infestation, moldiness, or other forms of decomposition.

Canned Vegetables

Canned vegetable products must be prepared from sound, wholesome raw materials free from decomposition. Definitions and standards of identity for a wide variety of canned vegetables provide that "the food is processed by heat, in an appropriate manner, before or after being sealed in a container so as to prevent spoilage." The importance of adequate heat processing of canned vegetables, particularly the nonacid types, is emphasized by the special regulations for low-acid canned foods.

Cans of food which have become swollen or otherwise abnormal are adulterated and should be destroyed.

Standards of quality have been promulgated for many vegetables. These are minimum standards only and establish specifications for quality factors such as tenderness, color, and freedom from defects. If the food does not meet these standards, it must be labeled in bold type "Below Standard in Quality" followed by the statement "Good Food—Not High Grade," or a statement showing in what respect the product fails to meet the standard, such as "excessively broken," or "excessive peel" (21 CFR 130.14). The standards of quality for canned vegetables supplement the identity standards. In other words, the identity standards define what the product is and set floors and ceilings on important ingredients, while the quality standards provide for special labeling for any product which is not up to the usual expectations of the consumer but is nevertheless a wholesome food.

If a *fill-of-container* standard has not been promulgated for a canned vegetable, the container must nevertheless be well filled with the vegetable, with only enough packing medium to fill the interstices. In the case of canned tomatoes, no added water is needed or permitted.

The standards of fill for canned tomatoes and canned corn require that the solid food and the liquid packing medium occupy not less than 90% of the total capacity of the container. The standard for canned corn also specifies a minimum drained weight of 50% of the water capacity of the container for the solid corn ingredient. Canned mushrooms must meet minimum drained weight requirements, stated in ounces, for various can sizes; and canned green peas and field peas must comply with volumetric fill requirements which state that if the peas and liquid packing medium are poured from the container and returned thereto, the leveled peas (irrespective of the liquid) completely fill the container.

Shippers of *tomato products* (canned tomatoes, tomato juice, paste, puree, and catsup) should consult the standards of identity for these items (21 CFR 155.190–4). Attention is called to the salt-free tomato solids requirements for puree and paste and to the fact that neither artificial color nor preservatives is permitted in any of these products. Tomato juice is unconcentrated; tomato puree must contain not less than 8%, and tomato paste not less than 24% salt-free tomato solids.

These tomato products are occasionally contaminated with rot because of failure to remove decayed tomatoes from the raw material entering the cannery. Flies and worms are also filth contaminants of tomato products. The preparation of a clean tomato product requires proper washing, sorting, and trimming of the tomatoes and frequent cleaning of the cannery equipment, such as tables, utensils, vats, and pipelines.

In judging whether tomato products have been properly prepared to eliminate rot and decay, the Food and Drug Administration uses the Howard mold-count test and refuses admission to import shipments and takes action against domestic shipments if mold filaments are present in excess of amounts stated in the Food Defect Action Levels. Methods of testing tomato products are given in the *Official Methods of Analysis of the Association of Official Analytical Chemists*.

Dried Fruits and Vegetables

What has been said about preventing contamination of food applies particularly to perishable products such as dried fruit and vegetables, which are subject to attack by insects or animals or to deterioration resulting in moldiness or other forms of decomposition.

Dried Figs and Dates

Dried figs, both domestic and foreign, are subject to insect infestation during their growth and when stored under unsuitable conditions. Figs may also become moldy if not properly stored and handled. The industry has made substantial progress in eliminating conditions which result in contamination or spoilage of figs, but it is still necessary to refuse entry to some dried figs and fig paste because of insect or rodent contamination, mold, sourness, or fermentation.

Dried dates are refused entry if insect infested, if they contain other forms of filth, or if they are moldy or decomposed. The presence of unpitted dates or dates containing broken pieces of pits in shipments of "pitted dates" is also a cause of refusing shipments.

Dried Mushrooms

Only edible species of dried mushrooms may be offered for import. The most common bar to entry, however, is insect infestation, usually by flies or maggots. Dried wild mushrooms should be handled by people who know how to sort out insect-infested mushrooms and those not clearly identifiable as edible species. If insect infestation is so heavy in a particular growing area that it is impractical to sort out the insect-infested ones, then the mushrooms from that area should not be offered for entry. The mushrooms should be protected during drying and storage to prevent their contamination with insects, rodent and bird filth, or other objectionable material. Canned mushrooms should be essentially free of insect infestation. Since the canned product is prepared from domesticated varieties grown under enclosure, the careful producer can readily prevent access by insects.

Fresh Fruits

Apples and other fruits bearing excessive residues from insecticide sprays or dusts are adulterated under the federal law. (See the next section entitled "Pesticidal Residues on Raw Agricultural Commodities.")

Pineapples showing or likely to show the internal condition known as "brown heart" or "black heart" should not be offered for entry into the United States.

Blueberries and huckleberries sometimes contain small larvae which render them unfit for food. Fruit from infested areas should be avoided. Fresh blueberries should be held and transported under conditions which will prevent mold or other types of spoilage.

Pesticidal Residues on Raw Agricultural Commodities

"Raw agricultural commodity" means any food in its raw or natural state, including all unprocessed fruits, vegetables, nuts, and grains. Foods that have been washed, colored, waxed, or otherwise treated in their unpeeled natural form are considered to be unprocessed. Products of this kind containing pesticide residues are in violation of the Federal Food, Drug, and Cosmetic act unless: (1) the pesticide chemical has been exempted from the requirement of a residue tolerance; or (2) a tolerance has been established for the particular pesticide on the specific food and the residue does not exceed the tolerance (408).

Processed foods that contain any residue of a pesticide which is not exempted or for which no tolerance has been established are adulterated under section 402(a)(2)(C) of the Act. If a tolerance has been established, a pesticide residue in the processed food does not adulterate the ready-to-eat food if the residue does not exceed the tolerance established for the raw agricultural commodity. The applicable regulations are in 21 CFR 180 and 193.

Tolerances for pesticidal residues on many raw agricultural commodities have been established under section 408 of the law. Tolerances are established, revoked, or changed, as the facts warrant such action, by the Environmental Protection Agency. Firms considering offering for entry into the United States foods which may contain pesticidal residues should write to the Food and Drug Administration, Division of Regulatory Guidance (HFF-314), 200 C Street S.W., Washington, D.C. 20204, for current information concerning the enforcement of tolerances for residues on raw agricultural products.

Fruit Jams (Preserves), Jellies, Fruit Butters, Marmalades

The standards of identity for jams and jellies were revised in 1974. The revised standards (21 CFR 150) require that these products be prepared by mixing not less than 45 parts by weight of certain specified fruits (or fruit juice in the case of jelly) and 47 parts by weight of other designated fruits to each 55 parts by weight of sugar or other optional nutritive carbohydrate sweetening ingredient. Only sufficient pectin may be added to jams and jellies to compensate for a deficiency, if any, of the natural pectin content of the particular fruit. The standards also require that for both jams (preserves) and jellies the finished product must be concentrated to not less than 65% soluble solids.

Standards of identity have also been established for artificially sweetened jams and jellies, and for these products the fruit ingredient must be not less than 55% by weight of the finished food product.

The standard of identity for fruit butters was revised in 1975. Fruit butters are defined as the smooth, semisolid foods made from not less than five parts by weight of fruit ingredient to each two parts by weight of sweetening ingredient. As is the case with jams and jellies, only sufficient pectin may be added to compensate for a deficiency, if any, of the natural pectin content of the particular fruit. The fruit butter standard requires that the finished product must be concentrated to not less than 43% soluble solids.

There is no formal standard of identity for citrus marmalade. However, the FDA expects a product labeled sweet orange marmalade to be prepared by mixing at least 30 pounds of fruit (peel and juice) to each 70 pounds sweetening ingredients. Sour or bitter (seville) orange marmalade, lemon marmalade, and lime marmalade would be prepared by mixing at least 25 pounds of fruit (peel and juice) to each 75 pounds of sweetening ingredient. The amount of peel should not be in excess of the amounts normally associated with fruit. The product should be concentrated to not less than 65% soluble solids. Such products would not be regarded as misbranded.

Jams, jellies, and similar fruit products should, of course, be prepared only from sound fruit. Decayed or decomposed fruits and insect-contaminated fruits should be sorted out and discarded.

Confectionery (Candy)

The utmost in cleanliness and sanitation should govern the manufacture of confectionery, because both the raw materials and the finished products tend to attract rodents and insects. Stored materials should be inspected frequently and carefully. Equipment should be washed thoroughly and kept free from accumulation of materials that would attract vermin.

The presence of nonpermitted colors and misbranding by the incorrect listing of ingredients also constitutes grounds for detentions or seizure. Fruit-type confectionery containing any artificial fruit flavor must be labeled as "artificially flavored" in the manner specified by the regulations [21 CFR 101.22(i)(2)].

Nonnutritive objects with the exception of such objects that are of practical functional value to the confectionery product and do not render the product injurious or hazardous to health, and alcohol other than that from flavoring extracts not in excess of 0.5% are specifically prohibited in confectionery.

Manufacturers who use colors should make sure these colors are authorized for use in the United States, and, if they require certification, that they are from a batch certified as suitable for use in foods by the U.S. Food and Drug Administration.

Cocoa Products

Standards of identity have been promulgated under the Federal Food, Drug, and Cosmetic Act for approximately 40 cacao products. If a cacao product is labeled as one of the standardized products listed in the regulations, the shipper or buyer should take care to ensure that it conforms to the standard for that product (21 CFR 163).

Excess shell is frequently the cause of detention of various standardized cacao products.

Cocoa beans offered for import sometimes show damage which bars them from entry. Beans with mold permeating the bean or showing clouds of spores when cracked are objectionable, as are wormy, insect-infested beans which may show live or dead insects, webbing, or insect excreta. Moldy and insect-infested beans should be removed from the lot before shipment. Care should be taken to store beans before and during shipment so that mold and insect contamination are prevented. Some shipments have been encountered which contained animal excretia—evidence of storage or handling under unsanitary conditions.

Beverages and Beverage Materials

Alcoholic Beverages

Beer, wines, liquors, and other alcoholic beverages are specifically subject to the Federal Alcohol Administration Act which is enforced by the Bureau of Alcohol, Tobacco and

Firearms of the U.S. Treasury Department. Accordingly, questions of labeling and of composition should be taken up with the Bureau rather than with the Food and Drug Administration. This is not the case for cooking wines or for certain other alcoholic beverages, such as diluted wine beverages and cider beverages having less than 7% alcohol by volume, which are solely within the jurisdiction of the FDA.

Questions dealing with the presence of deleterious substances in alcoholic beverages (such as excess fusel oil and excess aldehydes in whiskey; methyl alcohol in brandy; glass splinters from defective bottles; toxic ingredients, such as arsenic, lead, or fluorine, resulting from the spraying of the fruit used in wine manufacture; and residues of toxic clarifying substances) are also dealt with by the Food and Drug Administration, as are questions relating to sanitation and filth. The importation of absinth and any other liquors or liqueurs that contain an excess of *Artemisia absinthium* is prohibited.

Nonalcoholic Beverages

Products sold as fruit juices may be sweetened if the label states the presence of the added sugar or other wholesome, nutritive sweetening agent (saccharin is not a nutritive sweetening agent), but they should not contain added water.

Fruit juices should be manufactured only from clean, sound fruit, in clean equipment. Proper preparation involves thorough washing, sorting to remove wormy or spoiled fruit, and trimming. Flies should not come in contact with the fruit or equipment.

Fruit juice beverages containing added water are subject to all the requirements for nonstandard foods, particularly the use of a common or usual name (21 CFR 102.5). This must include a declaration of the percentage of any characterizing ingredient which has a material bearing on the price or consumer acceptance of the product. Diluted orange juice beverages are specifically required to have the percentage of juice expressed in increments of 5% (21 CFR 102.32).

Noncarbonated beverages containing no fruit or vegetable juice must be named as required by the regulation [102.5(a)] and if the label in any way suggests that fruit or vegetable juice is present there must be an added statement such as "contains no _____ juice," with the space filled in with the name of the fruit or vegetable indicated by the flavor, color, or labeling of the product.

Nonalcoholic carbonated beverages are subject to the standard for "soda water" (21 CFR 165.175). Caffeine from kola nut extract or other natural caffeine-containing extracts may be used in any soda water but not to exceed 0.02% by weight of the finished food. All optional ingredients are required to be declared on the label.

Bottled Waters

The FDA has established standards of quality for bottled drinking water (21 CFR 103.35). All bottled waters other than mineral waters must comply with these standards. It is anticipated that mineral waters, by their very nature, would exceed physical and chemical limits prescribed in the Bottled Drinking Water Standard and are therefore exempt from the standard. In no case, however, will the FDA permit the presence of any substance in bottled mineral water at any level deemed toxic.

The FDA has also established Current Good Manufacturing Practice Regulations for processing and bottling waters (21 CFR 129).

The listing on the labels of mineral waters of minerals which are present in insignificant amounts is misleading. Such a listing of ingredients may convey an impression of nutritional and/or therapeutic benefit not possessed by water. If nutritional or health claims are made in labeling, then the requirements of the nutritional labeling regulations apply. All bottled waters offered for import should be

1. Obtained from sources free from pollution.
2. Bottled or otherwise prepared for the market under

sanitary conditions, with special reference to the condition of the bottles or other containers and of their stoppers.

3. Free from microorganisms of the coliform group.
4. Of good sanitary quality when judged by the result of a bacteriological examination to determine the numbers of bacteria growing on gelatin at 20° C and on agar at 37° C.
5. Of good sanitary quality when judged by the results of a sanitary chemical analysis.

Some of the types of misbranding found on mineral water labels are

1. Objectionable therapeutic claims.
2. False and misleading statements other than therapeutic claims.
3. Label statement of analysis inaccurate or otherwise misleading.
4. Undeclared addition of salts, carbon dioxide, etc.
5. Labeling of artificially prepared waters as "mineral water."

Tea

Tea (*Thea sinensis*) is not only subject to the Federal Food, Drug, and Cosmetic Act but also to the Tea Importation act. Under the latter law, tea offered for entry must meet the standards of purity, quality, and fitness for consumption prescribed under the Act.

Beverages brewed from the leaves of other plants cannot properly be labeled as tea but should be labeled for what they are. For example, maté or matté, or the beverage prepared from it, should not be labeled unqualifiedly as tea or South American tea, since such names might mislead consumers in the United States who may not be familiar with the fact that it is an entirely different plant and beverage from the tea commonly sold in the United States. Like tea or coffee, maté may be mildly stimulating because of its caffeine content, but it should not be represented as capable of producing health, energy, endurance, or other physiological effects.

Coffee

Green coffee imported into the United States should be held at all times under sanitary conditions to prevent contamination by insects, rats, and mice.

The following conditions class coffee as objectionable and subject to refusal of entry: coffee berries which are black, part black, moldy, water damaged, insect eaten or infested, brown ("sour"), "Quakers" (immature berries), shriveled, "sailors," or those that contain foreign material such as pods, sticks, stones, trash, and "sweepings" of spilled coffee in ships' holds and on docks. Contamination by ores and other poisonous materials in the cargo also has resulted in detentions.

Fishery Products

Fish and shellfish are imported in the fresh, frozen, pickled, canned, salted, dried, or smoked conditions. The raw materials are by nature extremely perishable and must be handled rapidly under adequate refrigeration if decomposition is to be avoided. The conditions of handling are also likely to result in contamination unless particular safeguards are imposed.

Sometimes preservatives have been used to prevent or retard spoilage in fish. Any preservative used must be one accepted by FDA as safe and must be declared on the label.

Chemical contamination of lakes, rivers, and the oceans has been found to concentrate in certain species of fish. Excessive residues of pesticides, mercury, and other heavy metals are prohibited.

Names for Seafoods

To prevent substitution of one kind of seafood for another and consequent deception of the consumer, it is essential that labels bear names which accurately identify the products designated. Words like *fish*, *shellfish*, or *mollusk* are not sufficient; the name of the specific seafood must be used. Many fish, crustaceans, and mollusks have well-established common or usual names throughout the United States (for example, *pollock*, *cod*, *shrimp*, and *oyster*). These may not be replaced with other names, even though the other names may be used in some areas or countries. Neither may they be replaced with coined names, even though the coined names may be considered more attractive or to have greater sales appeal.

A more difficult problem is deciding what constitutes the proper designation for a seafood which has not previously been marketed in the United States and thus which has not acquired an established common or usual name in this country. In selecting an appropriate name for such a product, full consideration must be given to its proper biological classification and to avoiding a designation which duplicates or may be confused with the common or usual name in this country of some other species.

Labels on frozen fishery products for which no standards of quality have been promulgated need not make reference to quality, but if they do, the product must correspond to the usual understanding of the labeled grade. Particular care must be taken not to use the term "Grade A" on products that do not meet the established understanding of these terms in the United States.

Canned Fish

Canned fish generally are "low-acid canned foods" and packers are therefore subject to the registration requirements outlined on page 142.

Failure to declare the presence of added salt or the kinds of oil used as the packing medium in canned fish has resulted in the detention of fish products. If permitted artificial colors or chemical preservatives are used, their presence must be conspicuously declared in the labeling. Artificial coloring is not permitted if it conceals damage or inferiority or if it makes the product appear better or of greater value than it is.

The packing of canned fish and fish products with excessive amounts of packing medium has resulted in many detentions. If the fish are in a packing medium such as anchovies in oil, the container should be as full as possible of fish with the minimum amount of oil. The fact that the oil may be equal in value or even more expensive than the fish does not affect this principle. Canned lobster paste and similar products have been encountered which were deceptively packaged because of excessive headspace, that is, excessive space between the lid of the can and the surface of the food in the can.

Canned Pacific salmon is required to comply with standards of identity and fill of container. The standards establish the species and names required on labels and the permitted styles of pack (21 CFR 161.170).

Products represented as *anchovies* should consist of fish of the family *Engraulidae*. Other small fish, such as small herring and herringlike fish which may superficially resemble anchovies, cannot properly be labeled as anchovies. The product should be prepared from sound raw material and the salting or curing should be conducted in such a manner that spoilage does not occur.

The term *sardines* is permitted in the labeling of the canned products prepared from small-sized clupeoid fish. The sea herring (*Clupea Harengus*), the European pilchards (*Sardina pilchardus* or *Clupea pilchardus*), and the brisling or sprat (*Clupea sprattus*) are commonly packed in small-sized cans and labeled as sardines. The terms "brisling sardines" and "sild sardines" are permissible in the labeling of canned small brisling and herring, respectively. Large-sized herring cannot be labeled sardines. These canned products must be free from all forms of decomposition such as "feedy," "belly-blown" fish and must be adequately processed to prevent active spoilage by microorganisms. Fish are called "feedy fish" when their stomachs are filled with feed at the time the fish are taken from the water. Such fish deteriorate rapidly until the viscera and thin belly wall disintegrate, producing a characteristic ragged appearance called "belly-blown."

A standard of identity defines the species of fish that may be canned under the name *tuna* [21 CFR 161.190(a)]. There is also a standard for fill of container of canned tuna [21 CFR 161.190(c)]. The standards provide for various styles of pack, including solid pack, chunk or chunk style, flakes, and grated tuna. Provision is also made for various types of packing media, certain specified seasonings and flavorings, color designations, and methods for determining fill of containers.

The standard of fill of container for canned tuna specifies minimum values for weights of the pressed cake of canned tuna depending on the form of the tuna ingredient and the can size.

The canned fish *Sarda chilenis*, commonly known as the bonito or bonita, may not be labeled as tuna since it is not a true tuna, but must be labeled as bonito or bonita. The fish *Seriola dorsalis*, commonly known as "yellowtail," must be labeled as yellowtail and may not be designated as tuna.

Fresh and Frozen Fish Fillets

These products are highly perishable and require extraordinary care if decomposition is to be avoided. The manufacturer must exercise extreme care in the selection of raw materials to remove any unfit, decomposed material and then to maintain the product in a sound, wholesome condition.

Shellfish Certification

Because raw shellfish—clams, mussels, and oysters—may transmit intestinal diseases such as typhoid fever, or be carriers of natural or chemical toxins, it is most important that they be obtained from unpolluted waters and produced, handled, and distributed in a sanitary manner.

Shellfish must comply with the general requirements of the federal Food, Drug, and Cosmetic Act and also with requirements of state health agencies cooperating in the National Shellfish Sanitation Program (NSSP) administered by the FDA and in the Interstate Shellfish Sanitation Conference (ISSC).

Shellfish harvesting is prohibited in areas contaminated by sewage or industrial wastes. To enforce this prohibition, these areas are patrolled and warning signs are posted by state health or fishery control agencies. State inspectors also check shellfish harvesting boats and shucking plants before issuing approval "certificates" which are equivalent to a state license to operate. Plants having approved certificates are required to place their certification number on each container or package of shellfish shipped. The number indicates the shipper is under state inspection and that he meets the requirements of the NSSP. It also serves the important purpose of identifying and tracing shipments found to be contaminated. Shippers are also required to keep records showing the origin and disposition of all shellfish handled and to make these records available to the control authorities.

Certain shellfish, particularly mussels and clams, may contain a naturally occurring marine toxin derived from plankton organisms upon which the shellfish feed. Such toxic shellfish may cause illness or even death. State shellfish control agencies also maintain surveillance of shellfish growing areas for marine biotoxins. The areas where these biotoxins periodically occur are from Maine to Massachusetts, Florida, and the west coast including Alaska.

Standards of identity have been set for raw oysters, Pacific oysters, and canned oysters. The standards define the sizes of oysters and prescribe the methods of washing and draining to prevent adulteration with excess water. A fill-of-container standard for canned oysters fixes the drained weight at not less than 59% of the water capacity of the container (21 CFR 161.130-161.145).

Shellfish Imports

Imported fresh and fresh frozen oysters, clams, and mussels are certified under the auspices of the National Shellfish Sanitation Program through bilateral agreements with the country of origin. Canada, Japan, the Republic of Korea, Iceland, Mexico, England, and New Zealand now have such agreements.

For further information on the requirements of the National Shellfish Sanitation Program write to: Food and Drug Administration, Shellfish Sanitation branch (HFF-344), 200 C Street S.W., Washington, D.C. 20204.

Caviar and Fish Roe

The name "caviar" unqualified may be applied only to the eggs of the sturgeon prepared by a special process. Fish roe prepared from the eggs of other varieties of fish, prepared by the special process for caviar, must be labeled to show the name of the fish from which they are prepared, for example, "whitefish caviar." If the product contains an artificial color, it must be an approved color and its presence must be stated on the label conspicuously. No artificial color should be used which makes the product appear to be better or of greater value than it is. If a chemical preservative is employed, it must be one approved by the FDA and it must be declared on the label.

Rock Lobster, Spiny Lobster, and Sea Crayfish

The sea crayfish, *Palinurus vulgaris*, is frequently imported into the United States in the form of frozen tails, frozen cooked meat, or canned meat. By long usage, the terms "rock lobster" and "spiny lobster" have been established as common or usual names for these products. No objection has been offered to either of these terms, providing the modifying words *rock* or *spiny* are used in direct connection with the word *lobster* in type of equal size and prominence.

In examination of imports, decomposition has sometimes been detected in all three forms of the product. In the canned product, decomposition resulted from the packing of decomposed raw material and also from active bacterial spoilage. In the frozen cooked products, detentions have been necessary also because of the presence of microorganisms indicative of pollution with human or animal filth as well as of decomposition.

Shrimp

Standards set minimum requirements for canned wet- and dry-pack shrimp and frozen raw breaded shrimp (21 CFR 161.173). This product must also comply with the regulations for low-acid canned foods.

Meat and Poultry

Meat and Meat Food Products

Meat or meat products derived from cattle, sheep, swine, goats, and horses are subject to the provisions of the Wholesome Meat Act enforced by the Food Safety and Inspection Service of the U.S. Department of Agriculture as well as certain provisions of the FDC Act. Foreign meat products must originate in countries whose meat inspection programs have been approved. Each shipment must be properly certified by the foreign country and upon inspection by the federal meat inspectors found to be completely sound, wholesome, and fit for human food before entry into the United States. Requests for inspection should be made to the Food Safety and Inspection Service, U.S. Department of Agriculture, Washington, D.C. 20250. The imported product after admission into the United States becomes a domestic article subject not only to the Federal Meat Inspection Act but also to the Federal Food, Drug, and Cosmetic Act to the extent the provisions of the Meat Inspection Act do not apply. Wild game, however, is subject to the requirements of the Federal Food, Drug, and Cosmetic Act and its regulations.

Poultry and Poultry Products

Poultry and poultry products offered for importation are subject to the Wholesome Poultry Act also enforced by the Food Safety and Inspection Service, to which inquiries concerning such products should be addressed. The term "poultry" means any live or slaughtered domesticated bird (chickens, turkeys, ducks, geese, or guineas), and the term "poultry product" means any poultry which has been slaughtered for human food, from which the blood, feathers, feet, head, and viscera have been removed in accordance with rules and regulations promulgated by the Secretary of Agriculture, or any edible part of poultry, or, unless exempted by the Secretary, any human food product consisting of any edible part of poultry, separately or in combination with other ingredients.

Poultry and poultry products are also subject to the Federal Food, Drug, and Cosmetic Act to the extent to which the provisions of the Poultry Products Inspection Act do not apply.

Soups generally are under the jurisdiction of the U.S.D.A. However, those containing small amounts of cooked meat, poultry, or broth as flavoring ingredients are subject to regulation by the FDA.

Gelatin

Gelatin is not held to be a meat food product amenable to the Federal Imported Meat Act. The provisions of the Food, Drug, and Cosmetic Act require it to be prepared from clean, sound, wholesome, raw materials, handled under sanitary conditions. Gelatin should not contain glue or other gelatinlike material with a low gelatinous characteristic, nor have a disagreeable odor or taste. It should be so prepared and marketed as to be free from spoilage, filth, or putridity. It should be free from such preservatives, metals, and salts of metals as may render its use injurious to health.

Diary Products

Milk, cream, and dairy products made from them offer ideal conditions for the growth and survival of microorganisms. It is essential that milk be obtained from animals free from diseases and that all materials used in manufactured diary products be handled under sanitary conditions at all times to prevent contamination with disease-producing and spoilage organisms. While pasteurization offers a considerable safeguard against disease transmission, contamination by workers suffering from disease, by rodents, or by unclean equipment or the addition of unpasteurized ingredients after pasteurization can create a serious health hazard. In a like manner, spoilage organisms, such as undesirable bacteria, yeasts, and molds capable of causing decomposition of the raw materials or of the finished products, may be contributed by unsanitary handling. Products prepared from decomposed raw materials, products undergoing active spoilage, or those contaminated with disease-producing organisms are adulterated and subject to legal action.

Milk Safety

A safe and wholesome supply of fresh milk and cream for the U.S. consumer is the objective of the Federal-State Milk Sanitation Program administered by the FDA through Interstate Milk Shippers (IMS) Agreements. In this program the producers of Grade A pasteurized milk are required to pass inspections and be rated by cooperating state agencies. The ratings appear in the "IMS List" published by the FDA and revised quarterly. The list is used by state authorities and milk buyers to assure the safety of milk shipped from other states.

Uniformity and adequacy of state milk production regulations is obtained through a model Pasteurized Milk Ordinance (PMO) developed and revised under FDA leadership. The PMO is the basis for the milk sanitation laws and regulations of 49 states, the District of Columbia, and over 2000 local communities.

Cream and Milk for Manufacturing

Cream and milk used for the manufacture of dairy products should be clean and free from decomposition and from residues of pesticides and drugs. It is important to keep the cream for as short a period as possible, in a clean place, and to use clean utensils in handling and processing. Dairymen are advised to use pesticides on cows and in dairy barns only as directed and to avoid feeds which carry pesticidal residues. When treating cows with drugs for mastitis or other diseases the milk should not be sold until after the recommended period following the end of dosage.

Nonfat Dry Milk

Nonfat dry milk is defined in a standard provided by Act of Congress on July 2, 1956, as follows: " . . . nonfat dry milk is the product resulting from the removal of fat and water from milk and contains the lactose, milk proteins, and milk minerals in the same relative proportions as in the fresh milk from which it is made. It contains not over 5 per centum by weight of moisture. The fat content is not over $1\frac{1}{2}$ per centum by weight unless otherwise indicated. The term 'milk,' when used herein, means sweet milk of cows."

In addition, a standard of identity has been established for nonfat dry milk, fortified with vitamins A and D.

Import Milk Act

In addition to being subject to the requirements of the Food, Drug, and Cosmetic Act, milk and cream (including sweetened condensed milk) offered for import into the continental United States are subject to another federal act, the Import Milk Act, enforced by the Food and Drug Administration. Such products may be imported only under permit after certain sanitary and other prerequisites have been fulfilled.

Butter

Butter is defined in the standard provided by Act of Congress of March 4, 1923, as follows:

> . . . "butter" shall be understood to mean the food product usually known as butter, and which is made exclusively from milk or cream or both, with or without common salt, and with or without

additional coloring matter, and containing not less than 80 per centum by weight of milk fat, all tolerances having been allowed for.

Butter is examined for evidence of the use of dirty cream or milk and for mold which indicates the use of decomposed cream. Chemical additives and artificial flavor are not permitted.

Cheese

Cheese may be contaminated with insect and rodent filth during the handling of the milk, during the manufacture of the cheese, or during storage. This must be guarded against. Particular care should be taken not to use milk which may be contaminated with pesticides from forage fed to the animals or carelessly used in barns. Large quantities of cheese have been detained because of such contamination.

Standards of identity have been promulgated for most natural cheeses, process cheeses, cheese foods, and cheese spreads (21 CFR 133). Where a standard has been adopted for a particular variety of cheese, all cheeses belonging to the variety must comply with the standard and be labeled with the name prescribed in the standard.

Most of the standards prescribe limits for moisture and for fat. A few natural cheeses are required to be made from pasteurized milk. Most, however, may be made from either raw milk or pasteurized milk. When made from raw milk they are required to be aged for 60 days or longer. The 60 days aging is for the purpose of increasing the safety of the cheese. Requirements for longer aging are made for cheeses which need long aging to develop the characteristics of the variety. Shippers of cheese and foods made of cheese should consult the FDA standards before making shipments to the United States.

Evaporated Milk, Sweetened Condensed Milk

Under the established standard of identity for evaporated milk (21 CFR 131.130), this product must contain not less than

165

7.5% milk fat and not less than 25.5% total milk solids. Sweetened condensed milk, for which a standard has also been established (21 CFR 131.120), must contain not less than 28% total milk solids and not less than 8.5% milk fat. Sweetened condensed milk is also subject to the Import Milk Act, but evaporated milk (which is sterilized by heat) is not.

Nuts and Nut Products

Nuts are adulterated if they are insect infested or insect damaged, moldy, rancid, or dirty. Empty or worthless unshelled nuts should be removed by careful hand sorting or by machinery.

Care should be taken to eliminate infested, dirty, moldy, or rancid nuts from the shipment. Conditions which may cause nuts to be refused admission are described below.

Insect infestation. Nuts are insect infested if they contain live or dead insects, whether larvae, pupae, or adults, or if they show definite evidence of insect feeding or cutting, or if insect excreta pellets are present.

Dirt. Nut meats may become dirty because of lack of cleanliness in cracking, sorting, and packaging.

Mold. Nut meats occasionally are moldy in the shell and bear fruiting mold or mold hyphae.

Rancidity. Nuts in this class have an abnormal flavor characterized by rancidity. Rancid nuts are frequently soft and have a yellow, dark, or oily appearance.

Extraneous material. Stems, shells, stones, excreta should not be present.

Defect action levels have been established for tree nuts. Deliberate mixing of good and bad lots to result in defects under these levels is prohibited even though the percentage of defects in the mixed lots is less than the defect action level.

Aflatoxin. The aflatoxins are a group of chemically related substances produced naturally by the growth of certain common molds. The aflatoxins, especially aflatoxin B_1, are highly toxic, primarily causing acute liver damage in exposed animals. Aflatoxin B_1 also exhibits highly potent cancer-producing properties in certain species of experimental animals. Studies of certain population groups reveal that the consumption of aflatoxin-containing foods is associated with liver cancer in humans.

The presence of aflatoxin in nuts and other products at levels above established action levels is a significant public health problem and is a basis for seizing or refusing imports of products containing it.

Bitter almonds. Because of their toxicity, bitter almonds may not be marketed in the United States for unrestricted use. Shipments of sweet almonds may not contain more than 5% of bitter almonds. Almond paste and pastes made from other kernels should contain less than 25 parts per million of hydrocyanic acid (HCN) naturally occurring in the kernels.

Nuts and nut meats must be prepared and stored under sanitary conditions to prevent contamination by insects, rodents, or other animals. Nuts imported for pressing of food oil must be just as clean and sound as nuts intended to be eaten as such or to be used in manufactured foods.

Standards for nut products. Mixed tree nuts, shelled nuts, and peanut butter are subject to FDA standards (21 CFR 164). The standards establish such factors as the proportions of various kinds of nuts and the label designations for "mixed nuts," the fill of container for shelled nuts, and the ingredients and labeling for peanut butter. All packers and shippers of nut products should be aware of the requirements of these standards.

Edible Oils

Olive oil is the edible oil expressed from the sound, mature fruit of the olive tree. Refined or extracted oil is not entitled to the unqualified name "olive oil." Other vegetable oils should be labeled by their common or usual name, such as cottonseed, sunflower, peanut, and sesame. Mixtures of edible oils should be labeled to show all the oils present and the names should be listed on the labels in the descending order of predominance in the product. The terms "vegetable oil" or "shortening" are not permitted to be used in food labeling without disclosing the source of each oil or fat used in the product (31 CFR 101.4(b)(14)]. Pictures, designs, or statements on the labeling must not be misleading as to the kind or amount of oils present or as to their origin.

Cod liver oil is a drug as well as a food since it is recognized in the *United States Pharmacopeia* (USP). Its value as a food, whether intended for human or animal use, depends mainly on its vitamin D content. Articles offered for entry as cod liver oil must comply with the identity standard prescribed by the USP and conform to the other specifications set forth in that official compendium.

Margarine, Mayonnaise, and Salad Dressings

Standards of identity have been established for margarine, mayonnaise, French dressing, and salad dressing. The margarine standard is in 21 CFR 166, and the standards for mayonnaise, French dressing, and salad dressing are in Part 169. There are also many nonstandard dressings, subject to the general food labeling requirements. Mineral oil is not a permitted ingredient in any of these foods (21 CFR 169).

Olives

Pitted and stuffed olives containing more than an unavoidable minimum of pits or pit fragments are regarded as in violation of the Food, Drug, and Cosmetic Act. While it may not be possible to completely eliminate this problem, dealers have been put on notice that they must take steps to reduce it to the extent that is reasonably feasible (see Food Defect Action Levels.

Spices, Seeds, and Herbs

This group includes food materials that particularly need protection from various animal and insect pests. They may also become moldy or otherwise decomposed unless properly prepared and stored. The U.S. food law requires emphasis on the principle of "clean" food, not "cleaned" food. One of the most serious consequences of failure to protect herbs and spices is contamination with excreta from rats, mice, birds, chickens, or other animals. Emphasis should be placed on harvesting, storing, handling, packing, and shipping under conditions which will *prevent* contamination.

The same basic principle of prevention applies in the case of insects. Gauze netting spread over foods drying in the open may be necessary to keep insects out of storage or packing places. Careful cleaning and fumigation of premises and equipment before a new crop is put into a storage space may save it from contamination by insects surviving from the previous crop. The use of infested secondhand bags is another common source of trouble.

While insecticides and fumigants have their function (for example, in preparing a storage space for spices or other foods), a product which is already infested is not made acceptable for food by fumigation. Insects are objectionable in food even though they may have been killed.

Most insecticides and fumigants are poisonous, and if they contaminate food, the food becomes adulterated and subject to legal action. While most fumigants are volatile, they may nevertheless result in contamination of the food or adversely affect nutritive values. Legal tolerances for such residues have been issued (21 CFR 193).

In some cases herbs or spices may be used for drug purposes and they then become subject to the drug provisions of the FDC Act. Those spices or spice oils which are in the *United States Pharmacopeia* or the *National Formulary* are subject to the standards set forth in these compendia when used for drug purposes.

Many herbs once thought to have medicinal value continue to be marketed for various purposes. If no therapeutic claims are made or implied in the labeling or other promotional material, such products are regarded as foods and subject only to the food provisions of the law. For example, the herb ginseng is permitted to be sold as a tea.

"Herbs" are not necessarily harmless, contrary to common beliefs. Many such plants are toxic and may be extremely dangerous. The Food and Drug Administration believes it important to prevent the marketing and use of herbs for medicinal purposes if they have not been determined to be safe and effective for their intended uses, as required by law.

Spices and herbs must be the genuine products indicated by their common names on the labels. If obtained from or mixed with material from other plants, they are both adulterated and misbranded. The identity of herbs and spices is established by their botanical names. For example, the herb labeled as "sage" is *Salvia officinalis* L. As a guide to *identity* of food spice products, the Food and Drug Administration uses the following definitions:

Spices Aromatic vegetable substances used for the seasoning of food. They are true to name, and from them no portion of any volatile oil or other flavoring principle has been removed. Onions, garlic, and celery are regarded as foods, not spices, even if dried.

Allspice The dried nearly ripe fruit of *Pimentia officinalis*, Lindl.

Anise The dried fruit of *Pimpinella anisum* L.

Bay Leaves The dried leaves of *Laurus nobilis* L.

Caraway Seed The dried fruit of *Carum carvi* L.

Cardamon The dried, nearly ripe fruit of *Elettaria cardamomum* Maton.

Cinnamon The dried bark of cultivated varieties of *Cinnamomum zeylanicum* Nees or of *C. cassia* (L.) Blume, from which the outer layers may or may not have been removed.

Ceylon Cinnamon The dried inner bark of cultivated varieties of *Cinnamomum zeylanicum* Nees.

Saigon Cinnamon, Cassia The dried bark of cultivated varieties of *Cinnamomum cassia* (L.) Blume.

Cloves The dried flower buds of *Caryophyllus aromaticus* L.

Coriander The dried fruit of *Coriandrum sativum* L.

Cumin Seed The dried fruit of *Cuminum cyminum* L.

Ginger The washed and dried, or decorticated and dried, rhizome of *Zingiber officinale* Roscoe.

Mace The dried arillus of *Myristica fragrans* Houtt.

Macassar Mace, Papua Mace The dried arillus of *Myristica argentea* Warb.

Marjoram, Leaf Marjoram The dried leaves, with or without a small proportion of the flowering tops, of *Marjorana hortensis* Moench.

Nutmeg The dried seed of *Myristica frangrans* Houtt, deprived of its testa, with or without a thin coating of lime (CaO).

Macassar Nutmeg, Papua Nutmeg, Male Nutmeg, Long Nutmeg The dried seed of *Myristica argentea* Warb, deprived of its testa.

Paprika The dried, ripe fruit of *Capsicum annuum* L.

Black Pepper The dried, immature berry of *Piper nigrum* L.

White Pepper The dried mature berry of *Piper nigrum* L. from which the outer coating or the outer and inner coatings have been removed.

Saffron The dried stigma of *Crocus sativus* L.

Sage The dried leaf of *Salvia officinalis* L.

Tarragon The dried leaves and flowering tops of *Artemisia dracunculus* L.

Thyme The dried leaves and flowering tops of *Thymus vulgaris* L.

Retail Food Protection

The FDA relies mainly on state and local authorities to ensure the safety of food passing through retail channels such as restaurants, cafeterias, supermarkets, snack bars, and vending machines. Given the size and diversity of the retail food industry, the FDA directs its efforts to promote effective state and local regulation. It assists and supports the development of model food protection laws and uniform standards by providing technical assistance, exchanging information, conducting training programs for regulatory personnel and, upon request, evaluating state programs.

Preventing the mishandling of food after it reaches the retailer is the primary concern of this joint federal/state effort. Foodborne disease has numerous causes, but results most often from improper holding and storage temperatures, inadequate cooking, poor hygienic practices by food handlers, and lack of cleanliness in facilities. Inquiries should be addressed to Retail Food Protection Branch (HFF-342), Food and Drug Administration, 200 C Street S.W., Washington, D.C. 20204.

Interstate Travel Sanitation

Sanitation requirements relating to passengers and crew on interstate carriers are contained in the regulations for Control of Communicable Diseases (21 CFR Part 1240) and Interstate Conveyance Sanitation (21 CFR Part 1250). These regulations contain specific requirements for equipment and operations for handling food, water, and waste both on conveyances (aircraft, buses, railroads, and vessels) and those located elsewhere (i.e., support facilities such as caterers and commissaries, watering points, and waste servicing areas). The regulations also specify requirements for reviewing plans and inspecting construction of equipment, conveyances, and support facilities. The carriers are required to use only equipment and support facilities which have been approved by the Agency.

For further information write: Food and Drug Administration, Division of Regulatory Guidance (HHF-312), 200 C Street S.W., Washington, D.C. 20204.

How To Obtain FDA Regulations

The Food and Drug Administration's regulations are published in the *Code of Federal Regulations* and are available in book format from the Government Printing Office. These books are revised each year as of April 1, to incorporate the revisions and additions from the previous year. The edition revised to April 1, 1988 may be purchased in single volumes or as a set as follows:

Title 21, CFR, Volume 1
    Parts 1 through 99
        General Regulations, Enforcement of the Act,
        Administrative Functions, Color Regulations

Title 21, CFR, Volume 2
    Parts 100 through 169
        Food Standards
        Special Dietary Foods, Good Manufacturing Practices
        for Foods, Thermally Processed Low-Acid Foods

Title 21, CFR, Volume 3
    Parts 170 through 199
        Food Additives

Title 21, CFR, Volume 4
    Parts 200 through 299
        General Drug Labeling Regulations, Restriction of Drug
        Manufacturers, Good Manufacturing Practices for Drugs

Title 21, CFR, Volume 5
    Parts 300 through 499
        Antibiotic Drugs, Investigational and New Drug
        Regulations

Title 21, CFR, Volume 6
    Parts 500 through 599
        Animal Drugs, Feeds, and Related Products

Title 21, CFR, Volume 7
    Parts 600 through 799
        Cosmetics, Biologics

Title 21, CFR, Volume 8
Parts 800 through 1299
Radiological Health, Medical Devices and
Miscellaneous Regulations

Title 21, CFR, Volume 9
Parts 1300 to End
Regulations of the Drug Enforcement Administration
and the Special Action Office for Drug Abuse
Prevention (Not FDA regulations.)

For prices and additional information contact the following:

Superintendent of Documents
Government Printing Office
Washington, D.C. 20402

List of FDA Offices and Addresses

FOOD AND DRUG ADMINISTRATION
5600 Fishers Lane
Rockville, MD, U.S.A. 20857
Regional and District Offices

Atlanta
880 West Peachtree, N.W.
Atlanta, GA 30309

Baltimore
900 Madison Avenue
Baltimore, MD 21201

Boston
585 Commercial Street
Boston, MA 02109

Buffalo
599 Delaware Avenue
Buffalo, NY 14202

Chicago
1222 Post Office Building
433 West Van Buren Street
Chicago, IL 60607

Cincinnati
1141 Central Parkway
Cincinnati, OH 45202

Dallas
3032 Bryan Street
Dallas, TX 75204

Denver
500 U.S. Customhouse
Denver, CO 80202

Detroit
1560 East Jefferson Avenue
Detroit, MI 48207

Kansas City
1009 Cherry Street
Kansas City, MO 64106

Los Angeles
1521 West Pico Boulevard
Los Angeles, CA 90015

Minneapolis
240 Hennepin Avenue
Minneapolis, MN 55401

Nashville
297 Plus Park Boulevard
Nashville, TN 37217

New Orleans
4298 Elysiana Fields Avenue
New Orleans, LA 70122

New York
850 Third Avenue
Brooklyn, NY 11232

Newark
20 Evergreen Place
East Orange, NJ 07018

Orlando
7200 Lake Ellenor Drive
Post Office Box 118
Orlando, FL 32802

Philadelphia
900 U.S. Customhouse
2nd & Chestnut Streets
Philadelphia, PA 19106

San Francisco
Room 526, Federal Office
Building
San Francisco, CA 94102

San Juan
Room 107, Post Office and
Courthouse Building
Post Office Box S-4427
San Juan, PR 00905

Seattle
909 First Avenue
Seattle, WA 98104

International communications may be expedited by sending them to:

International Affairs Staff (HFC-40)
Food and Drug Administration
Rockville, MD, U.S.A. 20857
Phone: (301) 443-4480

CHAPTER 7

Marketing Your Product

At this stage in your product development, the subject of marketing plays a very key role once again. In Chapter 1, we discussed the types of market research necessary to identify your product's consumer acceptability. In this chapter we are going to discuss marketing as it relates to your sales activities. Sales and marketing seem very similar; in fact, in most smaller companies they are handled by the same person and/or department. Actually, they are quite separate entities. Marketing is considered to be all the activity, research, and preparation necessary to present your product, at its best, to potential buyers. Sales is the activity which actually closes the deal.

Marketing Budget

It must be stressed that it is vitally important that you develop a marketing budget. It is essential that you develop goals and objectives for long-range planning as well as short-term results. When you have established your objectives and developed the strategies to achieve them, your marketing budget will specify how much it will cost and exactly how much you will have to spend.

When you are figuring your marketing budget, keep in mind that total marketing costs are usually a collection of all costs needed to get your food product into the hands of the consumer immediately (during market launch) and in the future. You need to organize your budget into specific categories such as sales, advertising, research, media relations, and community contributions. By organizing the marketing functions into specific categories, you can then put your money into those areas that match your goals and objectives. You can divide your budget (more here, less there) among those activities that satisfy short-term needs while allocating budget dollars for long-term strategies. If you take time to develop your budget in this way, you will have a much better chance of reaching your goal of success.

Appendix 1 at the end of this chapter is a list of various nationwide organizations, associations, and publications that can be helpful in developing your marketing strategies. Get in touch with some of these groups. Read. Educate yourself. Everything you will be developing for your particular product has been done before. Learn from your business peers. They would be happy to share their experiences and knowledge with you. There is a real spirit of "we're in this thing together" in the community of food processors, particularly among the small business owners. Get out there and get involved.

Distribution

Establishing the best method for distributing your product or finding the most advantageous channel of distribution for a processed food item can be somewhat tricky. A great deal depends on the volumes you can produce, the amount of promotional support (dollars) you have, and what market niche your product fits into.

The major channel of distribution for any food item is, of course, the grocery chains. To enter this channel, you can either sell direct or work through a broker or distributor. Selling direct can be tricky because fewer and fewer grocery buyers are willing to spare the time and energy meeting with the multitude of small, regional processors who want them to shelf their products. Your best bet is to get a reputable broker or distributor to handle your product for you.

The food industry is extremely competitive and becoming more so every year. In 1987, over 10,000 new products were launched and less than 1% were still on the market in January of 1989. Thousands of food products are competing for every inch of supermarket shelf space. It is important to plan an aggressive, yet well-thought-out strategy for your product. Food distributors and food brokers are the professionals who can help you compete.

A distributor sells your product directly to the stores. He has an established network of supermarket buyers that he regularly visits and sells to. A good distributor will act as both a sales and distribution force for your product. He will usually represent complementary, but not competitive, food products.

The major difference between a food distributor and a food broker is that the broker doesn't buy the product from you, while the distributor does. A broker never takes title to the product. He is simply a sales agent who sells your product for you. Depending on the type of product you are producing, you can expect a food broker to charge between 5 and 10% of total sales. Brokers usually handle a much larger portfolio of products. If your product falls into a mainstream category, such as dry grocery, deli, frozen food, or beverage, you ought to seriously consider a broker. Grocery store buyers often prefer the convenience of working with brokers to fill standard food slots.

Brokers and distributors are listed in the yellow pages of your phone book. Call some local food processors and find out which ones have the best reputation in your area. If you have a specialty food item, you probably want to consider a specialty food distributor. A distributor charges a larger percentage for services, sometimes as much as 25% if he is offering you full service. He will be able to handle all aspects of your sales and distribution, including freight. The freight service is no small matter, particularly if your processing facility happens to be located on a dirt road in the middle of the Rocky Mountains.

Distributors will put extra effort into working with new food processors. Another advantage is that a food distributor does take title to the goods and that can help your cash-flow position.

Many entrepreneur food processors feel that they can handle the sales and distribution elements of their business themselves. This may be possible in the very beginning stages of your business, but will it be worth the time and effort it will take from your other responsibilities? If your pricing structure is developed properly in the beginning, the cost of a broker, distributor, or some type of sales agent should be included. If you are going to market your product effectively, you will need to have an external sales force to assist you. To adequately cover a metropolitan area, you would need an internal sales force of 2 to 3 people. It would take from 25 to 30 persons on staff to geographically cover your national market. Do yourself a favor. Hire a good broker or distributor.

Another service provided by the broker or distributor is the monitoring of your product on the retail shelf. He will make sure that your product is in the right place, with the right number of slots (facings), and at the correct price. The bottom line is that buyers in the grocery industry like to deal with people they know. Hiring an established broker or distributor can be your best investment.

When hiring a broker or distributor, you must be prepared to give up a percentage of your profit for their services. These professionals, especially the best ones, are very choosy about the products they will represent, and there are so many food products coming on the market daily that they can afford to be selective. You will be expected to make a sales presentation to the broker or distributor. Be as prepared for this meeting as you would be for a typical sales call. You will have to convince your potential representative that he should handle your product for you. Do you have a break-through product, or new packaging, or better pricing? In the standard-sized grocery store there are over 16,000 products offered. In order for your product to be given a spot, someone else's product is going to have to be dropped. Your broker or distributor is going to have to convince the grocery buyer that your product will sell better and make more money than the competition, and you have to convince your broker or distributor that he can do that with your product.

Put a sales kit together. You will use a sales kit whenever you make sales presentations for your product. A sales kit includes company history, product information, and promotional support that you plan to use during the next year to move your product. Promotional support can include advertising, store samples, and deals or coupons that will be offered.

Whatever you do, be honest with your broker or distributor. Let him do his job. Deliver what you promise, work with him, and you will all benefit. Figure 7.1 is an excellent flowchart that will help identify your best available avenues of distribution.

Another good channel of distribution, and one often overlooked by food processors, is the institution market. Your state and federal government facilities such as schools, hospitals, and jails are usually the largest bulk-packed food consumers. Government procurement of a wide variety of food items accounts for billions of dollars in food sales per year. Part of that money could be yours. The market potential is impressive, but before you get too excited, it is important to give serious consideration to this market and your production capabilities. You should answer the following questions:

1. Can you supply the volume this market requires?
2. How consistent is the demand? Is it seasonal? Can you work around peak and slack periods?
3. Can you package to meet strict requirements?
4. Can you maintain quality and still make a profit within the pricing requirements?

If you feel that this market has potential for your business, you need to find out who is in charge of procurement in your region. Contact your state's Department of Purchasing. Most states have staff who are there to assist local suppliers in servicing state procurement contracts.

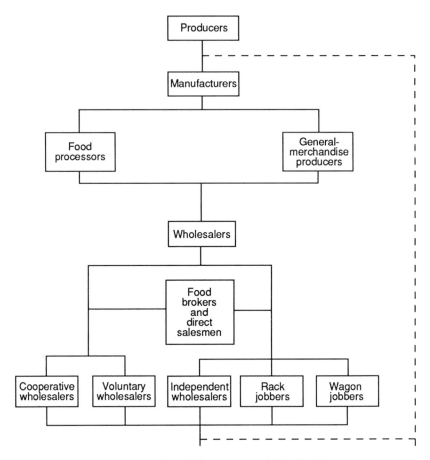

Figure 7.1   Available avenues of distribution.

Although the federal government does not make it easy for you (do they ever?), you can find out which agency and who you need to be talking with through various sources. The list of resources in Appendix 2 at the end of the chapter will assist you in obtaining valuable information on government procurement.

Small business owners interested in selling a food item to a federal agency may use a less formal process if they are planning on selling in small quantities. A small purchase ($10,000 or less) does not have to go through the formal solicitation and bid process. If you have made personal contact with a federal purchasing agent in your region, made a sales presentation, and he or she is interested in buying your product, you may sell directly to that agent. For small purchases, the purchasing agent has the option of asking for bids, selecting low bid, and dealing directly with the seller. If you win a bid, you will receive an official purchase order which, when signed by you, becomes your contract. Nothing to it!!

A very small food processor who is just beginning to tap his local market may wish to sell directly to individual grocery stores. Store managers may or may not support (and buy) locally produced and processed food. You will usually find willing buyers in the rural or suburban environs.

Sales Presentations

Although each grocery chain has its own set way of handling sales presentations, a listing of general requirements for supermarkets is given below so you can plan accordingly. You might want to talk to another local food processor who has already dealt with a particular buyer to obtain suggestions on how to conduct the presentation. This type of preparation will help you to make the best presentation possible and also help to build your confidence. A relaxed, confident presentation is your best sales tool!

Grocery and General Merchandise
Product Presentations

I. How to set an appointment with a supermarket merchandiser
A. Call the receptionist to determine the merchandiser responsible for the specific category.
B. Call 3–4 weeks in advance of desired appointment date.
C. Have the following paperwork completed before you meet with the merchandiser:

1. New-item form
2. Records of promotion allowance (RPAs): Outline of what kind of promotions (ads, coupons, in-store specials, etc.) have been done and are planned over the next 12 months.

II. Promotional support information you should have available when you meet with the merchandiser
   A. Television
     1. Which target area will be covered?
     2. What time slots? (Your broker will want to be sure that the time slots are appropriate for your target consumer):
       a. Morning hours and soap opera slots: Housewives
       b. 3:00–5:00: Children
       c. 9:00–12:00: Teens and young male adults
   B. Radio
     1. What stations?
     2. Why radio?
   C. Couponing
     1. Newspaper free-standing insert (FSI) (the 4-color multipage coupon magazine inserted into Sunday papers)
       a. How much is face value?
       b. How many lines?
       c. What newspaper?
     2. Magazines

III. Supermarket promotional programs
   A. Roto? (The advertising insert that grocery chains place in newspapers once a week, usually Wednesdays)
     1. ¼ page
     2. Oval
   B. Display monies available?
   C. Demo?
     1. How many stores?
     2. How often?

IV. Product distribution (New market entry?)
   A. Was this presented to us before?

B. Why did we turn down or discontinue?
C. Who carries this item?
D. What are specific area marketing information (SAMI) figures? (SAMIs are marketing figures that you buy from a private market research company.)
V. Product uniqueness
A. What need does this fulfill that is not already being met?
B. Who is your target market?
C. Are there similar products?
1. Why is your product different?
2. How will this expand category sales?
3. Different sizes?
D. Is there growth in this category?
VI. Test market
A. Where?
B. SAMI figures?
C. How does this compare to this market?
VII. Freight on board (FOB) pricing
A shipping term. Simply put it means the price quoted is to the buyer's workhouse. You pay for freight and handling costs, so build them into the price!

Meat Buying

I. Meat buying. All meat is bought centrally by one of our three meat buyers as follows:
A. Fresh beef. The buyer visits local packing plants and hand selects our beef needs in carcass form. This product is then shipped to our central meat plant for processing into primals for shipment to stores.
B. Fresh pork, lamb, and veal. The buyer contracts and buys all fresh meats by phone and/or by person-to-person meetings with local meat salesmen. This product is contracted for delivery the following week. Some items for special sale are contracted for up to 2 weeks in advance. All lamb is purchased from local producers.

C. Frozen and smoked meats. The buyer buys all meats by telephone or by person-to-person contact on an appointment basis. Most meats are purchased for delivery the following week. Some frozen items, such as turkeys, may be purchased up to 8 weeks prior to delivery.

II. Summary. Salespersons wishing to present new items and product lines must make an appointment with one of the buyers and present their products at the appointed time. All new products are then presented by the buyers to a central marketing committee meeting each Wednesday for approval. If the Committee approves the item it is then put into an order book as an authorized item.

Product Purchasing Outline

I. Prior to planting and production we will gladly arrange a time to discuss with each individual:
   A. Market history on specific items. Review standards.
   B. Needs we have experienced.
   C. Items we absolutely would not be able to buy from a new vendor.
   D. Payment and delivery expectations.
   E. Direct store delivery options.
II. After production is underway our field buyer will visit vendor facility and critique and compare to what is available elsewhere.
   A. Buy or reject based on supply/demand situation and quality considerations.
   B. Advise of current market prices and any expected changes.
   C. Arrange for direct store delivery if applicable and place orders throughout production cycle.

Trade Shows

No matter what channel of distribution or method of sales you decide upon, you should consider the excellent opportunity of exposing your product to potential buyers at a trade show. Trade shows are *very* big in the food industry. This section includes a list of food-industry trade shows held in 1989 just to give you an idea of the various sizes and numbers of shows available.

A trade show can offer you many opportunities to increase your product's visibility and sales. It is a good place to pick up new distributors and brokers. Often you will be asked to participate in a regional trade show in support of your distributor. As the following list indicates, trade shows run the gamut from small, locally sponsored tasting fairs, to the national Fancy Food Show held each year in New York City, to the enormous (half a million industry representatives in 1988) Food Show held each year in Tokyo, Japan. There are two wonderful publications that can be invaluable in helping you identify an appropriate show.

1. A book entitled *Trade Shows and Professional Exhibits Directory*. (updated annually.) It is published by Gale Research, Inc., Book Tower, Detroit, Michigan, 48226.
2. A weekly publication called *Tradeshow Week* is a magazine for and about the Tradeshow industry. The best feature is a master calendar of all U.S. and Canadian tradeshows that are scheduled between six months and one year from publication date. It is published by Tradeshow Week, Inc., 12233 W. Olympia Blvd., Suite 236, Los Angeles, California 90064-9956.

Either of these excellent publications should be available through your local business library or any of the state or local government agencies in your area working with small business.

There are several things to consider before choosing a particular show. You should contact the organizers of the show and ask them for specific information on the following.

1. Audience quality. It is important that the show audience include a very high percentage of actual buyers—the people in an organization who have the authority to make buying

decisions. It is nice to have the opportunity to talk to lots of people from a wide assortment of major companies, but if they can't authorize a buy you're wasting valuable sales time.

2. Audience size. A large audience is nice but it is imperative that the show organizers limit the attendees to trade only. Having the general public in to sample food products is basically the last "free lunch" program, and most small food processors can't afford it. The show organizers should have established a screening process to allow only buyers or trade people on the floor.

3. Promotional support. You should ask for specific information on how and where the organizers are going to promote the show. If it is not going to be advertised and promoted to your target market, obviously you could spend your time, money, and effort better at another show.

Another thing to determine when deciding on a show is the kind of support available through your state. Contact your state's Department of Agriculture and find out which shows its representatives are planning to attend or sponsor booths at. Most states have a trade show assistance program of one kind or another.

No matter what kind of show you decide to participate in, it will cost you time and money. Therefore, it is important that you prepare yourself and your staff adequately in order to maximize the benefits of the trade show.

If you are planning to participate in one of the major (high price tag) national or international shows, it is really wise to attend the show the year before you participate in order to "audit" the show. In other words, you don't have a booth, but you "work" the show to determine how it is organized, (sampling, etc.), how your competitors are presenting themselves, and where the best booths are located. This is also a good opportunity to make very preliminary contacts, which can be developed over the next 12 months and solidified at next year's show.

The following are a few common-sense tips for preparing for the trade show and for getting the most out of this special selling opportunity.

1. Develop a "lead card." Included below is a sample of a format that has worked well (see Box 7.1). Inserted in a 3-ring binder, the lead card keeps information organized during the show and helps make follow-up easier. Fill in as much of the information as you can while you are talking to your prospect. Record pertinent comments the moment he or she leaves. This will help you when you follow up on the lead days or weeks after the show.

2. Conduct preshow promotion if possible. Call present and potential customers. Send them a notice that you are going to have a booth at the show and invite them to stop by. If you can afford it and if the market warrants it, place an ad in the regional trade press. Include information about your product and where it can be seen and sampled.

3. Try to get *at least* one other qualified person to help you man the booth. It is important that this individual be qualified to answer questions about your product and provide specific product data, particularly sales numbers, volumes, etc. Choose someone who is capable of maintaining an enthusiastic attitude throughout the long hours of the show. Make sure you give yourself and your support staff time to relax away from the booth. This will keep you fresh and sharp. The most common booth schedule is 2 hours on and 2 hours off. When you and your sales staff are not working the booth, leave it! This keeps the booth clear and gives everyone time to unwind. Use this time to get something to eat. *Do not eat at your booth.* It projects a very unprofessional image!

4. Wear a badge or other identification (T-shirt, apron, etc.) with your product logo and your name. Remember, you have less than 5 minutes with each prospect, so sell yourself, your company, and your product.

5. Demonstrate and sample your product. If possible, involve prospects in the preparation and/or demonstration. Be confident and enthusiastic.

6. Pass out product samples and support materials sparingly. Give them only to prospects who demonstrate genuine interest and who have the authority to buy. Although most

BOX 7.1
LEAD CARD SAMPLE

Name: _____   Type of Business_____

Company: _____   Broker ☐

Address: _____   Distributor ☐

City/State: _____   Retailer ☐

Country: _____   Importer ☐

Telex or Fax: _____   Other _____

Telephone:_____   Other _____

Products interested in:_____
_____

What is the primary channel of distribution: _____
_____
_____
_____

Are you currently involved in import/export:_____

In what part of the country/world: _____

Specify products needed: _____
_____
_____
_____
_____

General Comments: _____
_____
_____
_____
_____

trade shows are industry only (closed to the general public), there are *always* people who walk around the show filling shopping bags in order to stock their pantries with free products. Don't give them the opportunity to have your product unless there is some real potential for a sale involved.

7. Finally, immediately following the show (within 72 hours), conduct a thorough follow-up with everyone involved with your booth. Ask yourself and your staff if your objectives were achieved and, if so, to what extent. If they were not met, ask yourselves what you did wrong and what could be done differently. Were you within budget? Did you attract a sufficient number of quality leads? Was your booth design appropriate? Was your product right for the show? Was the show right for your market goals? How well was your sales literature received? Are changes required? If so, what kinds of changes, and why?

If you generate at least ten healthy leads and learn from each show, any money spent on participating in a trade show is money well spent!

Transportation

Transportation costs are one of the most expensive components of the food industry, especially if your food processing facility is not located in or in proximity to a major urban market.

The average food processor has the choice of several different modes of freight—trucks, railroads, waterways, and airplanes. In the very early stages of their business developments, many food processors use companies such as United Parcel Service (UPS) or the U.S. mail parcel post to move small quantities of their product. This type of freight movement soon becomes costly and somewhat inefficient.

Transportation costs may limit the target market for your product. Shipping costs increase delivered costs, and this is what really effects your ability to compete on the shelf.

Until the 1980s the U.S. government had a great deal of control over the transportation industry. Routes were approved by the government, as were rates and services. Before deregulation of the industry, most carriers did not compete in price. Today you may find many different carriers or types (modes) of transportation competing for your freight business.

As a basic rule of thumb, you can expect to spend from 7 to 9 percent of your selling price for transportation costs. Nearly 75% of all freight is moved by trucks, at least part of the way between producer and consumer. Trucks have the bulk of short-haul cargo.

Although the majority of small food manufacturers use the trucking industry as their mode of transporting goods, several other alternatives are given below.

Water

In the United States, the inland waterways (like the Great Lakes and the Mississippi River) are used to transport bulky nonperishable products. This form of transportation is usually relatively inexpensive but is only available seasonally, as winter ice often closes freshwater harbors. Unless you are producing your food product very close to a freshwater harbor, this mode of transportation is not recommended. If your product is going overseas, however, ocean freight is usually the cheapest (but slowest) method of getting your product to your foreign buyer.

Air Freight

The most expensive cargo-transporting mode is the airplane. But, in rare instances, the greater speed may affect the added cost. Air freight created a new niche in the food industry by making fresh seafood available daily to consumers in land-locked areas. Tropical fruits, vegetables, and flowers (perishable commodities that simply could not be moved before) are now becoming familiar items on America's tables. Air freight is also important for small emergency or special-order shipments. Air freight should be considered when time is more important than price.

It should also be mentioned that some companies are using several different modes to move their food products. Often, a manufacturer will load its product on rail to be sent across country and then the product will be delivered to the whole-saler by truck. With the growing need for this kind of multi-mode cargo movement the "containerization" industry is really taking the lead. "Containerization" is the grouping of individual items into an economical shipping quantity and sealing them in protective containers for transit. This protects the product and simplifies handling during shipping. Some containers are as large as truck bodies.

This idea can also be carried further—"piggy back" services load truck tractors or flatbed trailers carrying containers on railcars to provide both speed and flexibility. Railroads now pick up truck trailers at the producer's location, load them onto specifically designed rail flatcars, and haul them as close to the customers as rail lines run. The trailers are then hooked up to truck tractors and delivered to the buyer's door.

Most transporting rates—the prices charged for cargo movement—are based on the idea that large quantities of a product can be shipped at a lower transport cost per pound than small quantities. Freight forwarders usually do not own their own transporting facilities, except perhaps for local delivery trucks. Rather, they wholesale air, ship, rail, and truck space. They accumulate small shipments from many shippers and reship in larger quantities to obtain lower transporting rates. "Common carriers" are basically involved in the same type of consolidation but more exclusively with the trucking mode.

Once your food processing business has outgrown UPS, parcel post, and/or personal delivery as reasonable freight options, it is important that you spend some time identifying what mode of transporting is most appropriate for your freight needs. Your local yellow pages will list the names of various freight company agents and representatives who would be happy to talk to you about rates and options. It is important to take the time educate yourself on your freight options because that cost can make the difference between success and failure.

Appendix 1

Food Dealers, Retail and Wholesale

Co-ops. Voluntary Chains and Wholesale Grocers. Annually. 1979. $86. Lists headquarters address, telephone number, number of accounts served, all branch operations, executives, buyers, annual sales volume (includes Canada and special "rack merchandiser" section). Chain Store Guide Publications, 425 Park Ave., New York, New York 10022.

Food Brokers Association, National Directory of Members. Annually in July. Free to business firms writing on their letterhead. Arranged by States and cities, lists member food brokers in the United States and Europe, giving names and addresses, products they handle, and services they perform. National Food Brokers Association, 1916 M St., N.W., Washington, D.C. 20036.

Food Service Distributors. Annually. 1979. $82. Lists headquarters address, telephone number, number of accounts served, branch operations, executives and buyers for distributors serving the restaurant and institutional market. Chain Store Guide Publications, 425 Park Ave., New York, New York 10022.

Fresh Fruit and Vegetable Dealers, The Blue Book of. Credit Book and Marketing Guide. Semiannually in April and October. (Kept up-to-date by weekly credit sheets and monthly supplements.) $225 a year. Lists shippers, buyers, jobbers, brokers, wholesale and retail grocers, importers, and exporters in the United States and Canada that handle fresh fruits and vegetables in carlot and trucklot quantities. Also lists truckers, truck brokers of exempt perishables with "customs and rules" covering both produce trading and truck transportation. Produce Reporter Co., 315 West Wesley St., Wheaton, Illinois 60187.

Frozen Food Fact Book and Directory. Annual. 1980. $50 to nonmembers, free to Association members. Lists packers, distributors, suppliers, refrigerated warehouses, wholesalers, and brokers; includes names and addresses of each firm and their key officials. Contains statistical marketing data. National Frozen Food Association, Inc., P.O. Box 398. 1 Chocolate Ave., Hershey, Pennsylvania 17033.

Grocery Register, Thomas'. Annual. 1979. 3 vols. $60/set. $45. Vol. 1 & 3 or Vol. 2 & 3. Volume 1: Lists supermarket chains, wholesalers, brokers, frozen food brokers, exporters, warehouses. Volume 2: Contains information on products and services; manufacturers, sources of supplies, importers. Volume 3: A–Z index of 56,000 companies. Also, a brand name/trademark index. Thomas Publishing Co., One Penn Plaza, New York, New York 10001.

Quick Frozen Foods Directory of Wholesale Distributors. Biannually. Lists distributors of frozen foods. Quick Frozen Foods, P.O. Box 6128, Duluth, Minnesota 55806.

Supermarket, Grocery & Convenience Store Chains. Annually. 1979. $97. Lists headquarters address, telephone number, location and type of unit, annual sales volume, executives and buyers, cartographic display of 267 Standard Metropolitan Statistical Areas (includes Canada). Chain Store Guide Publications, 425 Park Ave., New York, New York 10022.

Tea and Coffee Buyers' Guide, Ukers' International. Biennial. 1978–1979. Includes revised and updated lists of participants in the tea and coffee and allied trades. The Tea and Coffee Trade Journal, 18-15 Francis Lewis Blvd., Whitestone, New York 11357.

Restaurants

Restaurant Operators. (Chain). Annually, 1979. $94. Lists headquarters address, telephone number, number and location of units, trade names used, whether unit is company operated or franchised, executives and buyers, annual sales volume for chains of restaurants, cafeterias, drive-ins, hotel and motel food operators, industrial caterers, etc. Chain Store Guide Publications, 425 Park Ave., New York, New York 10022.

Manufacturers' Sales Representatives

Manufacturers & Agents National Association Directory of Members. Annually in July. $35 a copy—includes 12 monthly issues of Agency Sales. Contains individual listings of manufacturers' agents throughout the United States, Canada, and several foreign countries. Listings cross-referenced by alphabetical, geographical, and product classification. Manufacturers' Agents National Association, P.O. Box 16878, Irvine, California 92713.

Mass Merchandisers

Major Mass Market Merchandisers, Nationwide Director of. (Excludes New York Metropolitan area). Annually. 1980. $55. Lists men's, women's, and children's wear buyers who buy for over 175,000 units—top discount, variety, supermarket and drug chains; factory outlet stores; leased department operators. The Salesman's Guide, Inc., 1140 Broadway, New York, New York 10001.

Magazines and Trade Journals

Restaurants & Institutions
270 St. Paul Street
Denver, Colorado 80206-5191

Progressive Grocer
1351 Washington Blvd.
Stamford, Connecticut 06902

The Gourmet Retailer Magazine
1545 NE 123rd Street
North Miami, Florida 33161

Supermarket News (weekly newspaper)
P.O. Box 1400
Riverton, New Jersey 08077
(Wholesalers & brokers, $15/yr; others, $35/yr)

Food Trade News
119 Sibley Avenue
Ardmore, Pennsylvania 19003

Advertising Age
220 E. 42nd Street
New York, New York 10017

Ad Forum
18 E. 53rd Street
New York, New York 10022

ADWEEK
514 Shatto Place
Los Angeles, California 90020

Outlook
United Fresh Fruit &
  Vegetable Assn.
727 N. Washington Street
Alexandria, Virginia 22314

Food Production Management
2619 Maryland Avenue
Baltimore, Maryland 21218

Food Processing
301 E. Erie Street
Chicago, Illinois 60611

Prepared Foods
5725 E. River Road
Chicago, Illinois 60631

Food & Beverage Marketing
124 E. 40th Street
New York, New York 10016

Supermarket Business
Field Mark Media, Inc.
25 W. 43rd
New York, New York 10036
Shelby Report of the
  Southwest
1200 W. State Street
Garland, Texas 76040

Appendix 2

Federal Procurement

Federal Acquisition Regulation (FAR). Combined federal procurement regulations to be used by all agencies after April 1, 1984. Available from: Superintendent of Documents, U.S. Government Printing Office, Washington, D.C. 20402, (303) 844-3964. Cost: $143 for manual and 12–18 months of updates.

Commerce Business Daily. The *Commerce Business Daily* is published each working day by the Department of Commerce. The *CBD* lists all solicitations by civilian agencies estimated to be $10,000 or greater. It contains sections listing services and supplies. Each of these sections is further divided into specific types of service or supply. A number or alpha code is assigned to these specific categories. Services are assigned alpha codes; supplies, numeric. **Example:** Code J (service) pertains to "Maintenance and repair of equipment." Code 74 (supplies) is "Office machines." You can save time by learning the code of the supply/service you offer. You may subscribe to the *CBD* by writing the address below. Payment must accompany the order. Note: Many area libraries subscribe to the *CBD*. Available from: Superintendent of Documents, U.S. Government Printing Office, Washington, D.C. 20402, (202) 783-3238. Cost: Per year, $261 (first class) or $208 (fourth class). 6 months, $130 (first class) or $104 (fourth class)

Guide to Specifications and Standards of the Federal Government. This publication provides information on specifications and standards for products purchased by the U.S. Government, including "how government specifications and standards are developed and used," and "industry participation in the development of government specifications and standards." This publication is available at SBA offices. Cost: Free.

Product and Service Codes. Federal product and service codes are needed in completing bid forms. Available from: Federal Procurement Data Center, 4040 North Fairfax Drive, Arlington, VA 22203, (703) 235-1326.

Small Business Subcontracting Directory. Published by the Department of Defense, this publication contains company names and addresses of Department of Defense prime contractors by state and their small business liaison officer, product, or service line. Directory is published as an aid to small businesses seeking subcontracting opportunities. Available from: Superintendent of Documents, U.S. Government Printing Office, Washington, D.C. 20402. Cost: $7.

SBA Procurement and Technology Assistance. This 27-page booklet provides a brief explanation of how the federal government buys goods and services and of the legal provision for small businesses to participate in the procurement process. The booklet describes the bid process and several SBA resources which are available to assist small businesses: Procurement Automated Source System (PASS), and Certificate of Competency (COC) program. Available from: U.S. Small Business Administration. Cost: Free.

FPDC Standard Report. The standard report contains statistical procurement information in "snapshot" form for over 60 federal agencies as well as several other charts, graphs, and tables which compare procurement activities state by state, major product and service codes, method of procurement, and contractors. The report also includes quarterly and year-to-date breakdowns of amounts and percentages spent on small, women-owned, and minority businesses. Available from: Federal Procurement Data Center, 4040 North Fairfax Drive, Arlington VA 22203, (703) 235-1326. Cost: Free

Small Business and Government Research and Development. SBA book in Small Business Management Series, No. 28, includes a discussion of the procedures necessary to locate and sell to government agencies. Available from: Superintendent of Documents, U.S. Government Printing Office, Department 39-CC, Washington, D.C. 20402, (202) 783-3238.

Doing Business with the Federal Government. Principles and procedures of government procurement, government procurement programs, military procurement programs, general services administration procurement programs, other civilian agency procurement, government sales of surplus property, business services directory. Also available from Consumer Information Center, Department N, Pueblo, CO 81009. Available from: Superintendent of Documents, U.S. Government Printing Office, Washington, D.C. 20402, (202) 783-3238. Cost: $4.50.

"8(a)" Contracting. Through the 8(a) program small companies owned by socially and economically disadvantaged persons can obtain federal government contracts. The SBA acts as a prime contractor for selected federal government contracts and then awards those contracts to small companies in the 8(a) program. To be eligible for the 8(a) program, a business must be owned, controlled, and operated by one or more persons who are United States citizens and are determined by the SBA to be socially and economically disadvantaged. The business must be organized for profit and determined to

be small by SBA standards. By contacting the nearest SBA office, an 8(a) representative will furnish information concerning the program and explain the application process. The next step is preliminary counseling to determine feasibility of entering the program. Application forms are furnished the applicant if all the necessary requirements are met and sufficient contract support is available. Financial assistance in the form of loans, advance payments, and business development expenses are available to 8(a) program participants. These companies may be eligible to receive the bonding necessary to perform on government contracts. Available from: U.S. Small Business Administration.

Selling to the Military. This book provides information on locating sales opportunities for businesses with little or no experience in selling to the Department of Defense. Available from: Superintendent of Documents, U.S. Government Printing Office, Washington, D.C. 20402, (202) 783-3238. Cost: $8.

Small Business Accounting for Federal Government Contracts. This 5-page publication provides an overview of the types of compliance requirements small business owners are likely to face when entering government contract work. Sections cover sources of information on rules and regulations, important accounting issues, cost and pricing data requirements, governments audits, cost definitions, etc. Available from: Arthur Anderson & Co. Cost: Free to small business owners/operators.

CHAPTER 8

Looking to the Future— Exporting Your Product

The last thing you should consider as you are putting together your business strategy is the potential for overseas marketing of your product. Although it would be grossly premature for you to be including overseas marketing strategies in your start-up phase, there are some important things you can do (particularly in your packaging) that will save you time and money in the future should you decide to export your food product.

It is important to include on your packaging all weights and measurements in metric as well as standard English measurement. Most countries are already on the metric system and their standards for food and grocery products require the use of metric measurements.

Another very simple trick, but one that can make the difference between your product being exportable or not in many countries, is the addition of U.S.A. to the company address which appears on your packaging. An example of an export-ready label would be:

Manufactured by XYZ Company
100 Main Street
Compton, Colorado 10010
U.S.A.

If you would like to consider future international expansion, or if your food processing operation is up and running and you are looking toward developing a strong 3-year exporting plan, there are some things that you need to know. Keep in mind that all the following information is very general and there is a great deal of time and effort involved in successfully launching your product into international markets. The questions that follow have been found to be beneficial in helping business, specifically upper management, identify its readiness for exporting.

1. Is your company currently operating at or near capacity? The immediate profit potential from international sales will usually not offset expansion cost. Unless management is willing to carry these costs over 3 to 5 years, the profitability of international expansion may not be an attractive proposition.

2. Are you willing to modify your products and/or packaging to meet the requirements of foreign customers? Without exception, modifications of some kind will be necessary for each new market—from the relatively inexpensive translation of marketing materials and bilingualization of packaging to the extremely costly product modifications necessary to meet different standards. A commitment of up-front dollars is essential.

3. Do you have promotional literature that clearly describes your product's uses and methods of preparation? Are you willing to bear the expense of having this literature available in several languages? Again, an initial investment of funds must be committed to prepare your marketing materials for your sales launch.

4. Does your product require special handling? Is it sensitive to spoilage? Does it require extra packing before shipping? Special handling and freight cost can add enough to your price of goods to make it noncompetitive. Short shelf life of certain products makes them extremely poor candidates for successful overseas sales. Extra packaging cost must be added into pricing structure. These additional costs must be considered and can create an unreasonably high product price.

5. If you were to export, do you feel your product would be sensitive to any of the following factors?

Strong competition. Can you compete? Are you successfully competing against your domestic competition?

Changes in technology. Particularly with high-tech products, swift and effective market penetration is essential, costly, and carries a high risk.

Fashion or consumer preference. Market launch without extensive market research can be fatal.

Government policy. Fighting a government restriction or protective position is cost prohibitive to most companies, and an extremely long-term proposition.

Trademark infringement. This issue should be considered in preliminary strategy because attempting to deal with an infringement after the fact is prohibitively expensive and will dilute your product launch in all areas.

6. How would you feel about using a foreign representative or agent to sell your products or to represent your company's name in foreign markets? Entrepreneurs seem to have a hard time relinquishing control, especially to a foreign representative. Identifying a competent, well-connected sales representative overseas is often the key to success.

7. Which of the following factors has the strongest influence over your pricing strategy?

Profit margin. The flexibility of a wide profit margin is necessary because of all the additional costs involved in international trade.

Labor costs. Your product will probably be competing against products produced in low labor cost areas. Labor-sensitive products produced in the U.S. may not be able to compete.

Promotion and marketing costs. Promotion and marketing costs will be your major up-front expense in your overseas launch.

Competitors' prices. If you have the ability to maintain a competitive price, the chance of success is greatly increased when coupled with sufficient marketing dollars.

8. Is your product unique or of particularly high quality? If it isn't you should identify your special niche, because without one you probably shouldn't consider overseas expansion.

9. What percentage of your cost production is made up of labor costs? Ten percent? Twenty-five percent? Fifty percent? If labor costs are too high, you probably can't compete due to the low labor costs of your competitor's offshore production.

10. Is your product or business sensitive to seasonal fluctuations or other types of cycles? This can be worked to your advantage. Windows of opportunity, well used, can be your niche and, along with increased revenues due to new international sales channels, can make domestic operation more effective by stabilizing production and providing for more efficient capacity management. For example, a hot beverage will sell during winter months. Australia's seasons are opposite those of the United States. Your hot beverage product would probably sell well in that seasonal niche.

11. Which of the following would you rate as most important to your company: growth, stability, high return, security, or industry reputation? Stability, high return, and security are not words often associated with international business. If these are crucial to you, you would probably be happier sticking to domestic expansion.

12. Which term best describes the activity of your business over the past 3 years: robust, active, sustained, slacking, depressed, or volatile? International expansion should never be used in a "bail-out" situation. A strong revenue base is a must for successful international market expansion.

13. Which best describes your firm's strategy: high margin, market sensitive, high volume, or low volume? Again, flexibility in pricing structure, high up-front cost with potential for long-term profitability, must be seriously considered.

14. Has your firm ever worked jointly with another company on a product, or has your company ever worked as part of a team in providing services or other support to a project? This kind of managerial or corporate experience is invaluable in the global arena. It should be sought when staff expansion is feasible.

15. Are you able, and would you be willing, to extend credit or offer other financial terms to facilitate your entry into

a foreign market? Innovative finance packaging and credit terms designed to offset strength of the dollar (particularly when dealing in high-inflation economies) can give you a strong competitive edge, but companies should proceed with caution and secure payment through one of several federally supported insurance programs.

16. Are you willing and, without putting stress on other operations, able to invest in developing foreign markets even if it takes 2 years to recoup your investment and realize any profit? Aside from the fact that most international sales will be carried as receivable for an average of 60 to 90 days (which needs to be figured into your original pricing structure), the additional related costs of doing business overseas may negate profits for a substantially longer period than the average domestic transaction. Are you willing to listen to the constant moaning of your controller, credit manager, and accounting personnel?

17. How would management characterize exporting in relation to current operations: extension of existing activity, a new activity, a separate activity? Commitment of management is imperative. A strategy must be developed *and* accepted by all the key players. Lack of support or change of direction midstream will guarantee failure.

18. Which would you cite as the best reason for investing time, money, and effort to initiate an export marketing plan: to combat foreign competition, extend product life cycle, offset seasonal fluctuations, combat U.S. competitors, or distribute fixed costs over higher volumes? Each of these issues carries strong advantages to a company's growth and must be addressed in your preliminary strategy.

19. Have you identified a particular foreign market that you feel holds promise for your product? Would sales and marketing be handled in-house? Both questions must be answered in preliminary preparations. The cost of trained professional assistance at this stage is money well spent.

20. Which of the following do you consider to be the *greatest* obstacle preventing you from exporting: inadequate information and expertise, competition, unacceptable risks, or

unavailable financing? Each of these obstacles will make you noncompetitive. Congratulate yourself for taking a sensible look at your export capabilities and, if you're still committed to international expansion, start looking toward major reorganization and development.

The following matrix (Figure 8.1) is a very simplified explanation of some of the various channels of distribution available for your product. It is important to do a great deal of market research on the importing country and the industry niche of your product before you decide on any one of these distribution channels.

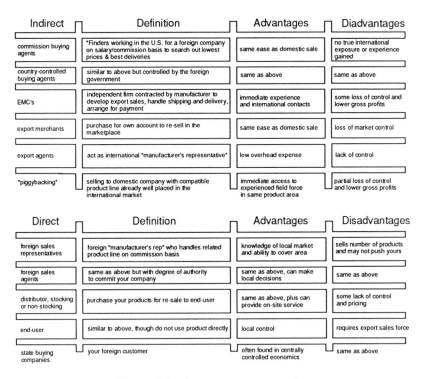

Figure 8.1   An export entry matrix.

At the end of the chapter is a glossary of basic international business terms that you will need to become familiar with if you are serious about overseas market expansion.

Remember, doing business overseas is not difficult, it's just different. No one is born understanding the logistics of an international transaction—it's a learning process.

Every state has at least one agency whose responsibility it is to assist small business owners in exploring international opportunities. Contact your state's international office—do *not* try to do international expansion alone! Appendix 1 is a list of various state agencies that can help you.

The following section is a summary of the excellent resources available to you through the federal government's International Trade Administration (ITA), which is an agency of the U.S. Department of Commerce. Appendix 2 is a list of all the International Trade Administration offices in the country. Contact the office in your state or region. They can be an enormous resource in helping you strategize potential international expansion.

Programs Offered by the International Trade Administration

Are you looking for international marketing tools and assistance that work? Then look to the U.S. and Foreign Commercial Service (US&FCS), an organization within the ITA of the U.S. Department of Commerce. Nowhere else can you find such a full line of high-quality products, programs, and services, as well as free one-on-one counseling by experts in the field of international trade.

Through the US&FCS, a U.S. firm has direct access to more than 95% of the global marketplace for U.S. products and services. Our U.S. offices are linked electronically to 124 overseas posts in 68 countries—a worldwide network of 1300 men and women dedicated to increasing the exports and profits of U.S. companies. The US&FCS is truly a global marketing arm for American business, especially valuable to the small and medium-sized business community which cannot afford direct representation in every potential market.

To find out what exporting is all about, start at your local district office, where a trade specialist will counsel you on an individual basis and walk you through the exporting process. Your trade specialist will help you identify your markets, assess these markets, find buyers and distributors overseas, and identify the most productive means for promoting your products.

The US&FCS has developed the trade strategies, information products, and programs that U.S. firms need for successful exporting. While all of the programs and services will not be suited to your specific needs, you should know all that the US&FCS is offering you. The following sections provide a detailed summary of these programs and services for your review.

Foreign Economic Trends

The economic trend reports pinpoint current and prospective economic and financial conditions and the marketing outlook for U.S. products. They are prepared by the American Embassy with contributions from commercial and economic staff. These reports are available for $1.00 each or on a subscription basis for $49/year from the Superintendent of Documents, U.S. Government Printing Office, Washington, D.C. 20402. Contact the District Office for individual country reports.

Foreign Buyer Program

The US&FCS has selected leading U.S. trade shows in industries with high export potential to participate in the Foreign Buyer Program. Through the Foreign Commercial Service employees, foreign buyers are encouraged to attend these shows. U.S. firms may participate in the shows in order to meet foreign buyers, agents/distributors, and potential licensees or joint-venture partners.

Market Identification and Assessment

Custom Statistics (U.S. Data, U.N. Data, U.N. Market Share Reports)

This material can be prepared on selected products or industries. Information which is available: statistics collected by the U.S. Bureau of Census, including export statistics and/or import statistics by commodity or country; United Nations export or import data; and Market Share Reports (MSRs), which identify the top world supplies of a given product. The time frames may be annual, quarterly, or monthly for the U.S. data, while only annual data is available for U.N. data. The reporting amounts may be by dollar value, quantity, unit value, or percentage of value or quantity. Costs vary from $10 to $750 depending on the amount of data needed and the complexity of the job; most reports are under $100.

Market Research Extracts

This research represents country and industry information which has been extracted and can be identified by product, country, and/or type of information. The extracts are currently being added to a centralized data base and will eventually include many categories. Currently eight industries are covered. A single extract includes a title, text, and bibliography. Pricing includes a $15 set-up charge plus $2 per abstract.

Comparison Shopping Service

A custom research service is offered for the following countries: Australia, Brazil, Canada, Colombia, France, Germany, India, Indonesia, Italy, Korea, Mexico, Philippines, Saudi Arabia, Singapore, and the U.K. Selected key marketing facts about a specific product will be researched in the particular country. Several basic questions will be answered: overall marketability;

names of key competitors; comparative prices; customary entry, distribution, competitive, and promotion practices; relevant trade barriers; names of potential agents or distributors, and potential licensing or joint-venture contacts. Fee for the service is $500 per country surveyed.

Market Contact Services

Agent/Distributor Service (ADS)

The Agent/Distributor Service (ADS) is designed to assist U.S. firms in locating potential agents, representatives, or distributors in foreign markets. This service is available on a worldwide basis (except in countries which conduct business through State Trading Agencies) at a cost of $125.00 per country or Canadian province. An ADS request is processed through the American Embassy or Foreign Service Post in the country involved, at which time contact is made with potential agents or distributors. The names and addresses of interested firms are sent to the requesting company through the Commerce District Office.

Computer Information Retrieval Service (CIRS)

This service makes available to U.S. businesses lists of foreign firms selected by electronic data processing techniques from automated files of compiled foreign commercial firms. These lists are tailored to fit individual requests, and printouts are available either on gummed mailing labels (with or without name of an officer contact) or in standard printout form with name and title of officer, year established, relative size, number of employees, date of information, and SIC product and/or service codes together with coding to indicate manufacturer, retailer, agent, etc.

The CIRS is a Lockheed DIALOG database which is accessible from the district office computer with printouts available in 2–5 days. Many files exist; the following are especially applicable for international trade:

1. Export mailing list (foreign trade index)
2. Trade opportunities, 1977 to present
3. Trade opportunities weekly, current 3 months

There is a $25 access charge; company's name and information are 25¢/listing, which includes all of the information listed above.

Commercial News

Commercial News USA is a magazine, published ten times per year, which provides worldwide advertising for U.S. products and services available for immediate export. This exposure enables foreign firms to identify and directly contact U.S. exporters, giving the U.S. company indications of market interest and often generating sales and agent contacts. The magazine is printed in a tissue-weight format, disseminated to U.S. Embassies, and thence mailed directly to interested parties in the respective country. Additionally, companies may choose to target selected world market areas (these have been divided into eight geographic groups), where special emphasis will be given to the product/service in these targeted areas.

Commercial News USA publishes seven issues, advertising products for selected industries as well as *new* products from all industries. Three issues are devoted to products from specific states or regions. To qualify for a new product ad, products must not have been sold on the U.S. market for more than 3 years. The Worldwide Services Program (WSP) notices are published in each issue. Service companies must have been doing business in the U.S. for at least 3 years in order to place an ad.

There is a variety of options on the size of advertisements:

Standard: $150   An ad with an 80-word listing and an optional photograph.

1/3 page: $400   This size and following sizes will include larger headlines, more detail, and more photographs, if provided.

2/3 page: $800
Full page: $1200
Two page: $3000
Cover 3: $2000

An additional $20.00/target area is optional.

World Traders Data Report Service (WTDR)

WTDRs are compiled by U.S. Foreign Service Officers and provide basic commercial and descriptive background information on individual foreign firms in selected countries as well as comprehensive information with respect to their commercial activities, competence, and reliability. If the WTDR information is not on file in Washington, it is requested by cable from the Foreign Commercial Service which responds by cable as soon as the information is developed. Cost is $100.00 per report.

Overseas Export Promotion

Matchmaker

Matchmakers are large, high-visibility trade delegations of top-level executives organized by the U.S. Department of Commerce. They help small and medium-sized U.S. firms develop export business with a minimal outlay of time and money. The events are held in selected countries and usually highlight specific products. The U.S. firms are "matched" with potential business partners in the host country in advance of the event. During the event, each company is set up in a booth where prescheduled, one-on-one interviews can be conducted in privacy.

U.S. Trade Center Shows

Permanent U.S. Trade Centers around the world are operated by the Department of Commerce to provide U.S. firms with opportunities to penetrate foreign markets by exhibiting their products to potential agents, distributors and buyers. Trade Centers provide year-round facilities for display and demonstration of U.S. products. An American firm with products fitting a particular show product theme may exhibit for a variable participation fee. The Trade Center staff conducts a widespread market promotion campaign, special trade showings, conferences, and press previews to attract importers, distributors, agents, buyers, and users to the exhibition.

International Trade Fairs

In addition to exhibitions held at the permanent overseas Trade Center, U.S. pavillions at international trade fairs offer manufacturers and representatives opportunities to display their products at trade fairs around the globe. If there are no trade fairs in a particular market, the U.S. Department of Commerce may arrange a solo exhibition (U.S. solo) of American products. The U.S. exhibitions at trade fairs overseas provide American firms with highly attractive, inviting, and functional exhibit areas at costs which vary from exhibition to exhibition but which are far less than it would cost firms to exhibit on their own.

Trade Missions

The Department of Commerce sponsors two types of Trade Missions—U.S. Specialized and Industry-Organized Government-Approved (IOGA)—which are highly effective overseas trade promotion techniques utilized by the Department of Commerce to expand U.S. exports. A trade mission's primary objectives are the sales of American-produced goods and services and the establishment of agencies and representatives abroad. *Specialized* missions are groupings of American companies with related products within given U.S. industry sectors to which the Department of Commerce provides both an Advance Officer and a Mission Director and arranges an overseas itinerary, business appointments, and receptions. All IOGA missions are organized and led by private export promotion organizations and receive substantial staff support from the Department of Commerce in the U.S. and abroad.

U.S. Catalog Exhibitions

Catalog exhibitions are overseas displays of American product catalogs, sales brochures, and similar graphic sales aids. They are designed to promote interest in and sales of American products abroad to help attract potential agents and distributors. They are staged as independent events, or in conjunction with trade shows, conferences, etc., usually in developing markets. A U.S. industry expert selected by the Department of Commerce represents the American industry and conducts lectures, plant visits, and panel discussions and prepares a market brief. Fee for U.S. firms varies, according to exhibition. Costs usually start around $75.00.

Video Catalog Exhibitions

Video catalog exhibitions are videotape presentations which take the place of live product demonstrations. The tapes enable the exhibitor to explain, demonstrate, and sell products more economically than could be done with a live exhibition. A U.S. industry technical representative is on hand to talk with potential buyers and answer their questions.

Between-Show Promotions

U.S. Trade Centers have occasional periods when the exhibit floor is not in use. U.S. companies, or their agents, may use the facilities at these times. Technical sales seminars are another form of product promotion which fit into between-show promotions. While U.S. firms do not receive the full range of services available to them at a trade exhibition, the commercial staff will counsel and assist in preparing for a successful promotion.

Miscellaneous

Major Projects

The Office of Major Projects provides assistance to U.S. firms in identifying foreign capital projects with major export potential. Firms are informed of these projects and may receive assistance in competing for the contracts. The service is free.

Business America

The Journal of International Trade. This is a top-notch business magazine geared toward a special interest—exporting. It is virtually an exporters' service. The magazine has articles on world trade outlooks by country, selected country coverage, and special industry studies. Also listed are trade leads, joint-venture opportunities, and licensing opportunities. Annual subscription fee is $40.

Overseas Business Reports

Country-specific marketing information is provided in these periodic reports. Included is information about channels of distribution, trade regulations, transportation, marketing practices, financing, investment, and industry trends. These reports are available on a subscription basis for $14/year from the Superintendent of Documents, U.S. Government Printing Office, Washington, D.C. 20402. Contact the District Office for individual country reports.

Conclusion

In this volume I have attempted to give you a lot of general information in as concise a format as possible to help you develop your strategy for a successful food processing operation.

It is absolutely *imperative* that you spend the necessary time, plan, do your marketing homework, and develop a strong business plan before you begin to spend a substantial amount of money.

Please take the time to locate the state, federal, and local agencies in your area which are in a position to help you, particularly during your development stages.

I wish you well in your endeavors and hope to see your name on the list of true American success stories! Kraft, Fields, Smuckers, Heinz, Del Monte, Dole, Contadina . . .

Glossary

Acceptance   This term has several related meanings, such as:

1. A time draft (or bill of exchange) which the drawee has accepted and is unconditionally obligated to pay at maturity. The draft must be presented first for acceptance—the drawee becomes the "acceptor"—then for payment. The word *accepted* and the date and place of payment must be written on the face of the draft.

2. The drawee's act in receiving a draft and thus entering into the obligation to pay its value at maturity.

3. (Broadly speaking) Any agreement to purchase goods under specified terms. An agreement to purchase goods at a stated price and under stated terms.

Ad valorem   According to value. See **Duty**.

Advance against documents   A loan made on the security of the documents covering the shipment.

Advising bank   A bank, operating in the exporter's country, that handles letters of credit for a foreign bank by notifying the exporter that the credit has been opened in his or her favor. The advising bank fully informs the exporter of the conditions of the letter of credit without necessarily bearing responsibility for payment.

Advisory capacity   A term indicating that a shipper's agent or representative is not empowered to make definitive decisions or adjustments without approval of the group or individual represented. Compare **Without reserve**.

Agent See **Foreign sales agent.**

Air waybill A bill of lading that covers both domestic and international flights transporting goods to a specified destination. This is a nonnegotiable instrument of air transport that serves as a receipt for the shipper, indicating that the carrier has accepted the goods listed and obligates itself to carry the consignment to the airport of destination according to specified conditions. Compare **Inland bill of lading, Ocean bill of lading,** and **Through bill of lading.**

Alongside A phrase referring to the side of a ship. Goods to be delivered "alongside" are to be placed on the dock or barge within reach of the transport ship's tackle so that they can be loaded aboard the ship.

Antidiversion clause See **Destination control statement.**

Arbitrage The process of buying Foreign exchange, stocks, bonds, and other commodities in one market and immediately selling them in another market at higher prices.

Asian dollars U.S. dollars deposited in Asia and the Pacific Basin. Compare **Eurodollars.**

ATA Carnet See **Carnet.**

Balance of trade The difference between a country's total imports and exports; if exports exceed imports, a favorable balance of trade exists; if not, a trade deficit is said to exist.

Barter Trade in which merchandise is exchanged directly for other merchandise without use of money. Barter is an important means of trade with countries using currency that is not readily convertible.

Beneficiary The person in whose favor a letter of credit is issued or a draft is drawn.

Bill of exchange See **Draft.**

Bill of lading A document that establishes the terms of a contract between a shipper and a transportation company under which freight is to be moved between specified points for a specified charge. Usually prepared by the shipper on forms issued by the carrier, it serves as a document of title, a contract of carriage, and a receipt for goods. Also see **Air waybill, Inland bill of lading, Ocean bill of lading,** and **Through bill of lading.**

Bonded warehouse A warehouse authorized by Customs authorities for storage of goods on which payment of Duties is deferred until the goods are removed.

Booking An arrangement with a steamship company for the acceptance and carriage of freight.

Buying agent See **Purchasing agent.**

Carnet A customs document permitting the holder to carry or send merchandise temporarily into certain foreign countries (for display, demonstration, or similar purposes) without paying duties or posting bonds.

Cash against documents (C.A.D.) Payment for goods in which a commission house or other intermediary transfers title documents to the buyer upon payment in cash.

Cash in advance (C.I.A.) Payment for goods in which the price is paid in full before shipment is made. This method is usually used only for small purchases or when the goods are built to order.

Cash with order (C.W.O.) Payment for goods in which the buyer pays when ordering and in which the transaction is binding on both parties.

Certificate of inspection A document certifying that merchandise (such as perishable goods) was in good condition immediately prior to its shipment.

Certificate of manufacture A statement (often notarized) in which a producer of goods certifies that manufacture has been completed and that the goods are now at the disposal of the buyer.

Certificate of origin A document, required by certain foreign countries for tariff purposes, certifying the country of origin of specified goods.

C & F "Cost and freight." A pricing term indicating that the cost of the goods and freight charges are included in the quoted price; the buyer arranges for and pays insurance.

Charter party A written contract, usually on a special form, between the owner of a vessel and a "charterer" who rents use of the vessel or a part of its freight space. The contract generally includes the freight rates and the ports involved in the transportation.

C & I "Cost and insurance" A pricing term indicating that the cost of the product and insurance are included in the quoted price. The buyer is responsible for freight to the named port of destination.

C.I.F. "Cost, insurance, freight." A pricing term indicating that the cost of the goods, insurance, and freight are included in the quoted price.

Clean bill of lading A receipt for goods issued by a carrier that indicates that the goods were received in "apparent good order and condition," without damages or other irregularities. Compare **Foul bill of lading**.

Clean draft A draft to which no documents have been attached.

Collection papers All documents (commercial invoices, bills of lading, etc.) submitted to a buyer for the purpose of receiving payment for a shipment.

Commercial attache The commerce expert on the diplomatic staff of his or her country's embassy or large consulate.

Commercial invoice An itemized list of goods shipped, usually included among an exporter's collection papers.

Commission agent See **Purchasing agent**.

Common carrier An individual, partnership, or corporation that transports persons or goods for compensation.

Confirmed letter of credit A letter of credit, issued by a foreign bank, with validity confirmed by a U.S. bank. An exporter who requires a confirmed letter of credit from the buyer is assured of payment by the U.S. bank even if the foreign buyer or the foreign bank defaults. See **Letter of credit**.

Consignment Delivery of merchandise from an exporter (the consignor) to an agent (the consignee) under agreement that the agent sell the merchandise for the account of the exporter. The consignor retains title to the goods until the consignee has sold them. The consignee sells the goods for commission and remits the net proceeds to the consignor.

Consular declaration   A formal statement, made to the consul of a foreign country, describing goods to be shipped.

Consular invoice   A document, required by some foreign countries, describing a shipment of goods and showing information such as the consignor, consignee, and value of the shipment. Certified by a consular official of the foreign country, it is used by the country's customs officials to verify the value, quantity, and nature of the shipment.

Convertible currency   A currency that can be bought and sold for other currencies at will.

Correspondent bank   A bank that, in its own country, handles the business of a foreign bank.

Countertrade   The sale of goods or services that are paid for in whole or in part by the transfer of goods or services from a foreign country. See **Barter**.

Credit risk insurance   Insurance designed to cover risks of nonpayment for delivered goods. Compare **Marine insurance**.

Customs   The authorities designated to collect duties levied by a country on imports and exports. The term also applies to the procedures involved in such collection.

Customhouse broker   An individual or firm licensed to enter and clear goods through customs.

Date draft   A draft that matures in a specified number of days after the date it is issued, without regard to the date of acceptance (definition 2). See **Draft**, **Sight draft**, and **Time draft**.

Deferred payment credit   Type of letter of credit providing for payment some time after presentation of shipping documents by exporter.

Demand draft   See **Sight draft**.

Destination control statement   Any of various statements that the U.S. government requires to be displayed on export shipments and that specify the destinations for which export of the shipment has been authorized.

Devaluation   The official lowering of the value of one country's currency in terms of one or more foreign currencies (e.g., if the U.S. dollar is devalued in relation to the French franc, one dollar will "buy" fewer francs than before).

DISC   Domestic international sales corporation.

Discrepancy, letter of credit   When documents presented do not conform to the letter of credit, it is referred to as a "discrepancy."

Dispatch   An amount paid by a vessel's operator to a charterer if loading or unloading is completed in less time than stipulated in the charter party.

Distributor   A foreign agent who sells for a supplier directly and maintains an inventory of the supplier's products.

Dock receipt   A receipt issued by an ocean carrier to acknowledge receipt of a shipment at the carrier's dock or warehouse facilities. Also see **Warehouse receipt**.

Documentary draft   A draft to which documents are attached.

Documents against acceptance (D/A)   Instructions given by a shipper to a bank indicating that documents transferring title to goods should be delivered to the buyer (or drawee) only upon the buyer's acceptance of the attached draft.

Draft (or Bill of exchange)   An unconditional order in writing from one person (the drawer) to another (the drawee), directing the drawee to pay a specified amount to a named drawer at a fixed or determinable future date. See **Date draft**, **Sight draft**, **Time draft**.

Drawback   Articles manufactured or produced in the United States with the use of imported components or raw materials and later exported are entitled to a refund of up to 99% of the duty charged on the imported components. The refund of duty is known as a "drawback."

Drawee   The individual or firm on whom a draft is drawn and who owes the stated amount. Compare **Drawer**. Also see **Draft**.

Drawer   The individual or firm that issues or signs a draft and thus stands to receive payment of the stated amount from the drawee. Compare **Drawee**. Also see **Draft**.

Dumping   Exporting/importing merchandise into a country below the costs incurred in production and shipment.

Duty   A tax imposed on imports by the customs authority of a country. Duties are generally based on the value of the goods (ad valorem duties), some other factor such as weight or quantity (specific duties), or a combination of value and other factors (compound duties).

EMC   See **Export management company**.

ETC   See **Export trading company**.

Eurodollars   U.S. dollars placed on deposit in banks outside the United States; usually refers to deposits in Europe.

Ex   "From." When used in pricing terms such as "Ex Factory" or "Ex Dock," it signifies that the price quoted applies only at the point of origin (in the two examples, at the seller's factory or a dock at the import point). In practice, this kind of quotation indicates that the seller agrees to place the goods at the disposal of the buyer at the specified place within a fixed period of time.

Exchange permit   A government permit sometimes required by the importer's government to enable the importer to convert his or her own country's currency into foreign currency with which to pay a seller in another country.

Exchange rate   The price of one currency in terms of another, i.e., the number of units of one currency that may be exchanged for one unit of another currency.

Eximbank   The Export–Import Bank of the United States.

Export broker   An individual or firm that brings together buyers and sellers for a fee but does not take part in actual sales transactions.

Export commission house An organization which, for a commission, acts as a purchasing agent for a foreign buyer.

Export declaration See **Shipper's export declaration**.

Export license A government document that permits the "Licensee" to engage in the export of designated goods to certain destinations. See **General export license** and **Validated export license**.

Export management company A private firm that serves as the export department for several manufacturers, soliciting and transacting export business on behalf of its clients in return for a commission, salary, or retainer plus commission.

Export trading company A firm similar or identical to an export management company.

F.A.S. "Free alongside." A pricing term indicating that the quoted price includes the cost of delivering the goods alongside a designated vessel.

FCIA Foreign credit insurance association.

F.I. "Free in." A pricing term indicating that the charterer of a vessel is responsible for the cost of loading and unloading goods from the vessel.

Floating policy See **Open insurance policy**.

F.O. "Free out." A pricing term indicating that the charterer of a vessel is responsible for the cost of loading goods from the vessel.

F.O.B. "Free on board." A pricing term indicating that the quoted price includes the cost of loading the goods into transport vessels at the specified place.

Force majeure The title of a standard clause in marine contracts exempting the parties for nonfulfillment of their obligations as a result of conditions beyond their control, such as earthquakes, floods, or war.

Foreign exchange The currency or credit instruments of a foreign country. Also, transactions involving purchase and/or sale of currencies.

Foreign freight forwarder See **Freight forwarder**.

Foreign sales agent An individual or firm that serves as the foreign representative of a domestic supplier and seeks sales abroad for the supplier.

Foreign trade zone See **Free trade zone**.

Foul bill of lading A receipt for goods issued by a carrier with an indication that the goods were damaged when received. Compare **Clean bill of lading**.

Free port An area such as a port city into which merchandise may legally be moved without payment of duties.

Free trade zone A port designated by the government of a country for duty-free entry of any nonprohibited goods. Merchandise may be stored, displayed, used for manufacturing, etc., within the zone and reexported without duties being paid. Duties are imposed on the merchandise (or items manufactured from the merchandise) only when the goods pass from the zone into an area of the country subject to the Customs Authority.

Freight forwarder An independent business which handles export shipments for compensation. (A freight forwarder is among the best sources of information and assistance on U.S. export regulations and documentation, shipping methods, and foreign import regulations.)

GATT "General Agreement on Tariffs and Trade." A multilateral treaty intended to help reduce trade barriers between the signatory countries and to promote trade through tariff concessions.

General export license Any of various export licenses covering export commodities for which validated export licenses are not required. No formal application or written authorization is needed to ship exports under a general export license.

Gross weight The full weight of a shipment, including goods and packaging. Compare **Tare weight**.

Import license A document required and issued by some national governments authorizing the importation of goods into their individual countries.

Inland bill of lading A bill of lading used in transporting goods overland to the exporter's international carrier. Although a through bill of lading can sometimes be used, it is usually necessary to prepare both an inland bill of lading and an ocean bill of lading for export shipments. Compare **Air waybill**, **Ocean bill of lading**, and **Through bill of lading**.

International freight forwarder See **Freight forwarder**.

IOGA Industry-organized, government-sponsored Trade Mission

Irrevocable letter of credit A letter of credit in which the specified payment is guaranteed by the bank if all terms and conditions are met by the drawee. Compare **Revocable letter of credit**.

Letter of credit (L/C) A document, issued by a bank per instructions by a buyer of goods, authorizing the seller to draw a specified sum of money under specified terms, usually the receipt by the bank of certain documents within a given time.

Licensing A business arrangement in which the manufacturer of a product (or a firm with proprietary rights over certain technology, trademarks, etc.) grants permission to some other group or individual to manufacture that product (or make use of that proprietary material) in return for specified royalties or other payment.

Manifest See **Ship's manifest**.

Marine insurance Insurance that compensates the owners of goods transported overseas in the event of loss that cannot be legally recovered from the carrier. Also covers air shipments. Compare **Credit risk insurance**.

Marking (or marks) Letters, numbers, and other symbols placed on cargo packages to facilitate identification.

Ocean bill of lading A bill of lading (B/L) indicating that the exporter consigns a shipment to an international carrier for transportation to a specified foreign market. Unlike an inland B/L, the ocean B/L also serves as a collection document. If it is a "straight" B/L, the foreign buyer can obtain the shipment from the carrier by simply showing proof of identity. If a "negotiable" B/L is used, the buyer must first pay for the goods, post a bond, or meet other conditions agreeable to the seller. Compare **Air waybill, Inland bill of lading,** and **Through bill of lading.**

On board bill of lading (B/L) A bill of lading in which a carrier certifies that goods have been placed on board a certain vessel.

Open account A trade arrangement in which goods are shipped to a foreign buyer without guarantee of payment. The obvious risk this method poses to the supplier makes it essential that the buyer's integrity be unquestionable.

Open insurance policy A marine insurance policy that applies to all shipments made by an exporter over a period of time rather than to one shipment only.

"Order" bill of lading (B/L) A negotiable bill of lading made out to the order of the shipper.

Packing list A list showing the number and kinds of items being shipped, as well as other information needed for transportation purposes.

Parcel post receipt The postal authorities' signed acknowledgment of delivery to receiver of a shipment made by parcel post.

PEFCO (Private Export Funding Corporation Lends to foreign buyers to finance exports from U.S.

Perils of the sea A marine insurance term used to designate heavy weather, stranding, lightning, collision, and sea water damage.

Phytosanitary Inspection Certificate A certificate, issued by the U.S. Department of Agriculture to satisfy import regulations for foreign countries, indicating that a U.S. shipment has been inspected and is free from harmful pests and plant diseases.

Political risk In export financing, the risk of loss due to such causes as currency inconvertibility, government action preventing entry of goods, expropriation or confiscation, war, etc.

Pro forma invoice An invoice provided by a supplier prior to the shipment of merchandise, informing the buyer of the kinds and quantities of goods to be sent, their value, and important specifications (weight, size, etc.).

Purchasing agent An agent who purchases goods in his or her own country on behalf of foreign importers such as government agencies and large private concerns.

Quota The quantity of goods of a specific kind that a country permits to be imported without restriction or imposition of additional duties.

Quotation An offer to sell goods at a started price and under specified conditions.

Remitting bank Bank that sends the draft to overseas bank for collection.

Representative See **Foreign sales agent.**

Revocable letter of credit A letter of credit that can be cancelled or altered by the drawee (buyer) after it has been issued by the drawee's bank. Compare **Irrevocable letter of credit.**

Schedule B Refers to "Schedule B, Statistical Classification of Domestic and Foreign Commodities Exported from the United States." All commodities exported from the United States must be assigned a 7-digit Schedule B number.

Shipper's export declaration A form required by the U.S. Treasury Department for all shipments and prepared by a shipper, indicating the value, weight, destination, and other basic information about an export shipment.

Ship's manifest An instrument in writing, signed by the captain of a ship, that lists the individual shipments constituting the ship's cargo.

Sight draft (S/D) A draft that is payable upon presentation to the drawee. Compare **Date draft, Time draft.**

Spot exchange The purchase or sale of foreign exchange for immediate delivery.

Standard Industrial Classification (SIC) A standard numerical code system used by the U.S. government to classify products and services.

Standard International Trade Classification (SITC) A standard numerical code system developed by the United Nations to classify commodities used in international trade.

Steamship conference A group of steamship operators that operate under mutually agreed upon freight rates.

Straight bill of lading A nonnegotiable bill of lading in which the goods are consigned directly to a named consignee.

Tare weight The weight of a container and packing materials without the weight of the goods it contains. Compare **Gross weight.**

Tenor (or a Draft) Designation of a payment as being due at sight, a given number of days after sight, or a given number of days after date.

Through bill of lading A single bill of lading converting both the domestic and the international carriage of an export shipment. An air waybill, for instance, is essentially a through bill of lading used for air shipments. Ocean shipments, on the other hand, usually require two separate documents—an inland bill of lading for domestic carriage and an ocean bill of lading for international carriage. Through bills of lading for international carriage. Through bills of lading are insufficient for ocean shipments. Compare **Air waybill, Inland bill of lading, Ocean bill of lading.**

Time draft A draft that matures either a certain number of days after acceptance or a certain number of days after the date of the draft. Compare **Date draft, Sight draft.**

Tramp steamer A ship not operating on regular routes or schedules.

Transaction statement A document that delineates the terms and conditions agreed upon between the importer and exporter.

Trust receipt Release of merchandise by a bank to a buyer in which the bank retains title to the merchandise. The buyer, who obtains the goods for manufacturing or sales purposes, is obligated to maintain the goods (or the proceeds from their sale) distinct from the remainder of his or her assets and to hold them ready for repossession by the bank.

Validated export license   A required document issued by the U.S. government authorizing the export of specific commodities. This license is for a specific transaction or time period in which the exporting is to take place. Compare **General export license**.

Warehouse receipt   A receipt issued by a warehouse listing goods received for storage.

Wharfage   A charge assessed by a pier or dock owner for handling incoming or outgoing cargo.

Without reserve   A term indicating that a shipper's agent or representative is empowered to make definitive decisions and adjustments abroad without approval of the group or individual represented. Compare **Advisory capacity**.

Appendix 1

State and Local Sources of Assistance

Alabama

U.S. Department of Commerce
US&FCS District Office
3rd Floor, Berry Building
2015 2nd Avenue North
Birmingham, Alabama 35203
(205) 254-1331

U.S. Small Business Administration
908 South 20th Street, Suite 202
Birmingham, Alabama 35205
(205) 254-1344

Alabama World Trade Association
777 Central Bank Building
Huntsville, Alabama 35801
(205) 539-8121

Office of International Trade
Department of Economic and
Community Affairs
P.O. Box 2939

Montgomery, Alabama 36105-0939
(205) 284-8721

Alaska

U.S. Department of Commerce
US&FCS District Office
701 C Street
P.O. Box 32
Anchorage, Alaska 99513
(907) 271-5041

U.S. Small Business Administration
701 C Street, Room 1068
Anchorage, Alaska 99501
(907) 271-4022

U.S. Small Business Administration
101 12th Avenue, Box 14
Fairbanks, Alaska 99701
(907) 452-0211

Alaska State Chamber of Commerce
310 Second Street
Juneau, Alaska 99801
(907) 586-2323

Anchorage Chamber of Commerce
415 F Street
Anchorage, Alaska 99501
(907) 272-2401

Department of Commerce and
Economic Development
Pouch D
Juneau, Alaska 99811
(907) 465-3580

Fairbanks Chamber of Commerce
First National Center
100 Cushman Street
Fairbanks, Alaska 99707
(907) 452-1105

Phoenix, Arizona 85003
(602) 254-5521

Director of International Trade
Office of Economic Planning and
Development
1700 W. Washington Street, Room 505
Phoenix, Arizona 85007
(602) 255-3737

Foreign Trade Zone No. 48
Papago Agency
P.O. Box 578
Sells, Arizona 85634
(602) 383-2611

Foreign Trade Zone No. 60
Border Industrial Development, Inc.
P.O. Box 578
Nogales, Arizona 85621
(602) 281-0600

Arizona

U.S. Department of Commerce
US&FCS District Office
Fed. Bldg. & U.S. Courthouse
230 N. 1st Ave., Rm. 3412
Phoenix, Arizona 85025
(602) 254-3285

U.S. Small Business Administration
3030 N. Central Avenue, Suite 1201
Phoenix, Arizona 85012
(602) 241-2200

U.S. Small Business Administration
301 W. Congress Street, Room 3V
Tucson, Arizona 85701
(602) 762-6715

Arizona World Trade Association
34 West Monroe, Suite 900

Arkansas

U.S. Department of Commerce
US&FCS District Office
320 West Capitol Avenue, Room 635
Little Rock, Arkansas 72201
(501) 378-5794

U.S. Small Business Administration
320 W. Capitol Avenue, Room 601
Little Rock, Arkansas 72201
(501) 378-5871

Arkansas Exporters Round Trade
1660 Union National Plaza
Little Rock, Arkansas 72201
(501) 375-5377

International Marketing
Department of Economic
Development

1 Capitol Mall
Little Rock, Arkansas 72201
(501) 371-7678

World Trade Club of Northeast
Arkansas
P.O. Box 2566
Jonesboro, Arkansas 72401
(501) 932-7550

California

U.S. Department of Commerce
US&FSC District Office
11777 San Vicente Boulevard,
Room 800
Los Angeles, California 90049
(213) 209-6707

U.S. Department of Commerce
US&FSC District Office
Federal Building, Room 15205
450 Golden Gate Avenue
Box 36013
San Francisco, California 94102
(415) 556-5860

U.S. Small Business Administration
2202 Monterey Street, Room 108
Fresno, California 93721
(209) 487-5189

U.S. Small Business Administration
350 South Figueroa Street, 6th Floor
Los Angeles, California 90071
(213) 688-2956

U.S. Small Business Administration
660 J Street, Room 215
Sacramento, California 95814
(916) 440-4461

U.S. Small Business Administration
880 Front Street, Room 4-S-29

San Diego, California 85701
(619) 293-5540

U.S. Small Business Administration
450 Golden Gate Avenue, Room 15307
San Francisco, California 94102

U.S. Small Business Administration
211 Main Street, 4th Floor
San Francisco, California 94105
(415) 556-0642

U.S. Small Business Administration
111 W. St. John Street, Room 424
San Jose, California 95113
(408) 275-7584

U.S. Small Business Administration
2700 N. Main Street, Room 400
Santa Ana, California 92701
(714) 836-2494

California State World Trade
Commission
1121 L Street, Suite 310
Sacramento, California 95814
(916) 324-5511

Department of Economic and
Business Development
1030 13th Street, Room 200
Sacramento, California 95814
(916) 322-1394

California Chamber of Commerce
International Trade Department
1027 10th Street
P.O. Box 1736
Sacramento, California 95808
(916) 444-6670

Century City Chamber of Commerce
International Business Council
2020 Avenue of the Stars, Plaza Level

Century City, California 90067
(213) 553-4062

Custom Brokers & Freight
Forwarders Association
303 World Trade Center
San Francisco, California 94111
(415) 982-7788

Economic Development Corporation
of Los Angeles County
1052 W. 6th Street, Suite 510
Los Angeles, California 90017
(213) 482-5222

Export Managers Association of
California
10919 Vanowen Street
North Hollywood, California 91605
(213) 985-1158

Foreign Trade Association of
Southern California
350 S. Figueroa Street, #226
Los Angeles, California 90071
(213) 627-0634

Inland International Trade
Association, Inc.
Bob Watson
World Trade Center
W. Sacramento, California 95691
(916) 371-8000

International Marketing Association
of Orange County
Cal State Fullerton
Marketing Department
Fullerton, California 92634
(714) 773-2223

Long Beach Area Chamber of
Commerce

International Business Association
50 Oceangate Plaza
Long Beach, California 90802
(213) 436-1251

Los Angeles Area Chamber of
Commerce
International Commerce Division
404 S. Bixel Street
Los Angeles, California 90017
(213) 629-0722

Los Angeles International Trade
Development Corporation
555 S. Flower Street, #2014
Los Angeles, California 90071
(213) 622-4832

Oakland World Trade Association
1939 Harrison Street
Oakland, California 94612
(415) 388-8829

San Diego Chamber of Commerce
101 West "C" Street
San Diego, California 92101
(619) 232-0124

San Francisco Chamber of Commerce
San Francisco World Trade
Association
465 California Street, 9th Floor
San Francisco, California 94104
(415) 392-4511

Santa Clara Valley World Trade
Association
P.O. Box 6178
San Jose, California 95150
(408) 998-7000

Valley International Trade
Association (San Fernando Valley)

1323 Carmelina Avenue, Suite 214
Los Angeles, California 90025
(213) 207-1802

World Trade Association of Orange
County
Hutton, 200 E. Sandpointe #480
Santa Ana, California 92707
(714) 549-8151

World Trade Association of
San Diego
P.O. Box 81404
San Diego, California 92138
(619) 298-6581

World Trade Council of
San Mateo Co.
4 West Fourth Avenue, Suite 501
San Mateo, California 94402
(415) 342-7278

Colorado

U.S. Department of Commerce
US&FCS District Office
U.S. Customhouse, Room 119
721 19th Street
Denver, Colorado 80202
(303) 837-3246

U.S. Small Business Administration
U.S. Customhouse, Room 407
721 19th Street
Denver, Colorado 80202
(303) 844-2607

Colorado Association of Commerce
and Industry
1390 Logan Street
Denver, Colorado 80202
(303) 831-7411

Denver Chamber of Commerce
1301 Welton Street
Denver, Colorado 80204
(303) 534-3211

Foreign Trade Office
Department of Commerce &
Development
1313 Sherman Street, Room 523
Denver, Colorado 80203
(303) 866-2205

Connecticut

U.S. Department of Commerce
US&FCS District Office
Federal Building, Room 610-B
450 Main Street
Hartford, Connecticut 06103
(203) 722-3530

U.S. Small Business Administration
One Hartford Square West
Hartford, Connecticut 06106
(203) 722-3600

International Division
Department of Economic
Development
210 Washington Street
Hartford, Connecticut 06106
(203) 566-3842

Delaware

U.S. Department of Commerce
US&FCS District Office
(See listing for Philadelphia,
Pennsylvania)

U.S. Small Business Administration
844 King Street, Room 5207

Wilmington, Delaware 19801
(302) 573-6294

Delaware State Chamber of
Commerce
One Commerce Center, Suite 200
Wilmington, Delaware 19801
(302) 655-7221

DelawareEastern Pennsylvania
Export Council
9448 Federal Building
600 Arch Street
Philadelphia, Pennsylvania 19106
(215) 597-2850

Division of Economic Development
Box 1401
630 State College Road
Dover, Delaware 19901
(302) 736-4271

Florida

U.S. Department of Commerce
US&FCS District Office
Federal Building, Suite 224
51 S.W. First Avenue
Miami, Florida 33130
(305) 350-5267

U.S. Small Business Administration
400 W. Bay Street, Room 261
Jacksonville, Florida 32202
(904) 791-3782

U.S. Small Business Administration
2222 Ponce de Leon Boulevard,
5th Floor
Miami, Florida 33134
(305) 350-5521

U.S. Small Business Administration
700 Twigs Street, Room 607

Tampa, Florida 33602
(813) 228-2594

U.S. Small Business Administration
550 45th Street, Suite 6
West Palm Beach, Florida 33407
(305) 689-2223

Bureau of International Trade and
Development
Department of Commerce
Collins Building
Tallahassee, Florida 32301
(904) 488-6124

Georgia

U.S. Department of Commerce
US&FCS District Office
1365 Peachtree Street, NE, Suite 504
Atlanta, Georgia 30309
(404) 881-7000

U.S. Department of Commerce
US&FCS District Office
Federal Building, Room A-107
120 Barnard Street
Savannah, Georgia 31401
(912) 944-4204

U.S. Small Business Administration
1720 Peachtree Road, N.W., 6th Floor
Atlanta, Georgia 30309
(404) 881-4749

U.S. Small Business Administration
52 North Main Street, Room 225
Statesboro, Georgia 30458
(912) 489-8719

Department of Industry and Trade
1400 N. OMNI International
Atlanta, Georgia 30303
(404) 656-3746

International Trade Division
Division of Marketing
Department of Agriculture
19 Martin Luther King, Jr., Drive
Atlanta, Georgia 30334
(404) 656-3600

Hawaii

U.S. Department of Commerce
US&FCS District Office
4106 Federal Building
300 Ala Moana Boulevard
P.O. Box 50026
Honolulu, Hawaii 96850
(808) 546-8694

U.S. Small Business
Administration
2213 Federal Building
300 Ala Moana Boulevard
Honolulu, Hawaii 96850
(808) 546-8950

Chamber of Commerce of Hawaii
World Trade Association
735 Bishop Street
Honolulu, Hawaii 96813
(808) 531-4111

Economic Development Corporation
of Honolulu
1001 Bishop Street
Suite 855, Pacific Tower
Honolulu, Hawaii 96813
(808) 545-4533

International Services Agency
Department of Planning & Economic
Development
P.O. Box 2359
Honolulu, Hawaii 96804
(808) 548-3048

Idaho

U.S. Department of Commerce
US&FCS District Office
(See listing for Salt Lake City, Utah)

U.S. Small Business Administration
1005 Main Street, 2nd Floor
Boise, Idaho 83701
(208) 334-1696

Division of Economic &
Community Affairs
Office of the Governor
State Capitol, Room 108
Boise, Idaho 83720
(208) 334-2470

Department of Agriculture
International Trade Division
120 Klotz Lane
P.O. Box 790
Boise, Idaho 83701

District Export Council
Statehouse, Room 225
Boise, Idaho 83720
(208) 334-2200

Idaho International Institute
1112 South Owyhee
Boise, Idaho 83705
(208) 342-4723

Idaho World Trade Association
Box 660
Twin Falls, Idaho 83301
(208) 326-5116

World Trade Committee
Greater Boise Chamber of Commerce
P.O. Box 2368
Boise, Idaho 83701
(208) 344-5515

Illinois

U.S. Department of Commerce
US&FCS District Office
Mid-Continental Plaza Building,
Room 1406
55 East Monroe Street
Chicago, Illinois 60603
(312) 353-4450

U.S. Small Business Administration
219 South Dearborn Street
Room 838
Chicago, Illinois 60604
(312) 886-0848

U.S. Small Business Administration
Four North, Old State Capitol Plaza
Springfield, Illinois 62701
(217) 492-4416

American Association of Exporters
and Importers
7763 S. Kedzie Avenue
Chicago, Illinois 60652
(312) 471-1958

Chamber of Commerce of Upper
Rock Island County
622 19th Street
Moline, Illinois 61265
(309) 762-3661

Chicago Association of Commerce
and Industry
World Trade Division
130 S. Michigan Avenue
Chicago, Illinois 60603
(312) 786-0111

Chicago Economic Development
Commission
International Business Division

20 N. Clark Street, 28th Floor
Chicago, Illinois 60602
(312) 744-8666

Customs Brokers and Foreign
Freight Forwarders Association of
Chicago, Inc.
P.O. Box 66365
Chicago, Illinois 60666
(312) 992-4100

Department of Commerce &
Community Affairs
International Business Division
310 South Michigan Avenue,
Suite 1000
Chicago, Illinois 60604
(312) 793-7164

Foreign Credit Insurance
Association
20 North Clark Street, Suite 910
Chicago, Illinois 60602
(312) 641-1915

Illinois Department of Agriculture
1010 Jorie Boulevard
Oak Brook, Illinois 60521
(312) 920-9256

Illinois Manufacturers' Association
175 West Jackson Blvd., Suite 1321
Chicago, Illinois 60604
(312) 922-6575

Illinois State Chamber of
Commerce
International Trade Division
20 N. Wacker Drive, Suite 1960
Chicago, Illinois 60606
(312) 372-7373

International Business Council
MidAmerica (IBCM)
401 North Wabash Avenue, Suite 538
Chicago, Illinois 60611
(312) 222-1424

Mid-America International Agri-
Trade Council (MIATCO)
300 West Washington Boulevard
Suite 1001
Chicago, Illinois 60606
(312) 368-4448

Northwest International Trade Club
P.O. Box 454
Elk Grove Village, Illinois 60007
(312) 793-2086

Overseas Sales & Marketing
Association of America, Inc.
3500 Devon Avenue
Lake Bluff, Illinois 60044
(312) 679-6070

Peoria Area Chamber of Commerce
230 SW. Adams Street
Peoria, Illinois 61602
(309) 676-0755

World Trade Club of Northern
Illinois
515 N. Court
Rockford, Illinois 61101
(815) 987-8100

Indiana

U.S. Department of Commerce
US&FCS District Office
One North Capitol
Indianapolis, Indiana 46204-2248
(317) 232-8846

U.S. Department of Commerce
US&FCS District Office
357 U.S. Courthouse & Federal
Office Building
46 East Ohio Street
Indianapolis, Indiana 46204
(317) 269-6214

U.S. Small Business Administration
575 N. Pennsylvania Street, Room 578
Indianapolis, Indiana 46204
(317) 269-7272

U.S. Small Business Administration
501 East Monroe Street, Room 160
South Bend, Indiana 46601
(219) 232-8361

Fort Wayne Chamber of Commerce
International Development Group
826 Ewing Street
Fort Wayne, Indiana 46802
(219) 434-1435

Greater Lafayette
Tippecanoe World Trade Council
Chamber of Commerce
P.O. Box 348
Lafayette, Indiana 47902
(317) 742-4041

Indiana Manufacturers Association
115 N. Pennsylvania Street, No. 950
Indianapolis, Indiana 46204
(317) 632-2474

Indiana State Chamber of Commerce
1 North Capitol, No. 200
Indianapolis, Indiana 46204
(317) 634-6407

Indianapolis Chamber of Commerce
Development and World Trade

320 N. Meridan
Indianapolis, Indiana 46204
(317) 267-2900

Indianapolis Economic Development
Corporation
48 Monument Circle
Indianapolis, Indiana 46204
(317) 236-6363

Michiana World Trade Club
230 W. Jefferson Blvd.
P.O. Box 1677
South Bend, Indiana 46634
(219) 234-0051

TransNational Business Club
College of Business
Ball State University
Muncie, Indiana 47306
(317) 285-5207

Tri State World Trade Council
329 Main Street
Evansville, Indiana 47708
(812) 425-8147

World Trade Club of Indiana, Inc.
P.O. Box 986
Indianapolis, Indiana 46206
(317) 261-1169

Iowa

U.S. Department of Commerce
US&FCS District Office
817 Federal Building
210 Walnut Street
Des Moines, Iowa 50309
(515) 284-4222

U.S. Small Business Administration
373 Collins Road, N.E.

Cedar Rapids, Iowa 52402
(319) 399-2571

U.S. Small Business
Administration
749 Federal Building
210 Walnut Street
Des Moines, Iowa 50309
(515) 284-4422

International Trade
Iowa Development Commission
600 East Court Avenue, Suite A
Des Moines, Iowa 50309
(515) 281-3581

Iowa Association of Business &
Industry
706 Employers Mutual Building
Des Moines, Iowa 50309
(515) 281-3138

Iowa–Illinois International Trade
Association
112 East Third Street
Davenport, Iowa 52801
(319) 322-1706

Siouxland Int. Trade Association
Legislative & Agriculture Affairs
101 Pierce Street
Sioux City, Iowa 51101
(712) 255-7903

Kansas

U.S. Department of Commerce
US&FCS District Office
(See listing for Kansas City,
Missouri)

U.S. Small Business Administration
110 East Waterman Street

234

Wichita, Kansas 67202
(316) 269-6571

Department of Economic
Development
International Trade Development
Division
503 Kansas Avenue, 6th Floor
Topeka, Kansas 66603
(913) 296-3483

International Trade Institute
1627 Anderson
Manhattan, Kansas 66502
(913) 532-6799

Kansas District Export Council
c/o Sunflower Manufacturing
Company
Box 628
Beloit, Kansas 67420
(913) 738-2261

Kentucky

U.S. Department of Commerce
US&FCS District Office
U.S. Post Office & Courthouse
Building, Room 636-B
Louisville, Kentucky 40202
(502) 582-5066

U.S. Small Business Administration
600 Federal Place, Room 188
Louisville, Kentucky 40201
(502) 582-5971

Kentuckiana World Commerce
Council
P.O. Box 58456
Louisville, Kentucky 40258
(502) 583-5551

Kentucky District Export Council
601 West Broadway, Room 636-B
Louisville, Kentucky 40202
(502) 583-5066

Louisville Economic Development
Cabinet
609 West Jefferson Street
Louisville, Kentucky 40201
(502) 586-3051

Office of International Marketing
Kentucky Commerce Cabinet
Capitol Plaza Tower, 24th Floor
Frankfort, Kentucky 40601
(502) 564-2170

TASKIT (Technical Assistance to
Stimulating Kentucky International
Trade)
College of Business and Economics
University of Kentucky
Lexington, Kentucky 40506-0205
(606) 257-7663

Louisiana

U.S. Department of Commerce
US&FCS District Office
432 International Trade Mart
2 Canal Street
New Orleans, Louisiana 70130
(504) 589-6546

U.S. Small Business Administration
1661 Canal Street, Suite 2000
New Orleans, Louisiana 70112
(504) 589-6685

U.S. Small Business Administration
500 Fannin Street
Room 6B14

Shreveport, Louisiana 71101
(318) 226-5196

Chamber of Commerce/New
Orleans and the River Region
301 Camp Street
New Orleans, Louisiana 70130
(504) 527-6900

Office of International Trade,
Finance and Development
Louisiana Department of Commerce
P.O. Box 44185
Baton Rouge, Louisiana 70804
(504) 342-5361

World Trade Club of Greater New
Orleans
1132 International Trade Mart
2 Canal Street
New Orleans, Louisiana 70130
(504) 525-7201

Maine

U.S. Department of Commerce
US&FCS District Office
(See listing for Boston,
Massachusetts)

U.S. Small Business Administration
40 Western Avenue, Room 512
Augusta, Maine 04333
(207) 622-8378

State Development Office
State House, Station 59
Augusta, Maine 04333
(207) 289-2656

Maryland

U.S. Department of Commerce
US&FCS District Office

415 U.S. Customhouse
Gay and Lombard Streets
Baltimore, Maryland 21202
(301) 962-3560

U.S. Small Business Administration
8600 La Salle Road, Room 630
Towson, Maryland 21204
(301) 962-4392

Baltimore Economic Development
Corporation
36 S. Charles Street, Suite 2400
Baltimore, Maryland 21201
(301) 837-9305

Division of Economic Development
45 Calvert Street
Annapolis, Maryland 21401
(301) 269-3944

The Export Club
326 N. Charles Street
Baltimore, Maryland 21201
(301) 727-8831

Massachussetts

U.S. Department of Commerce
US&FCS District Office
441 Stuart Street, 10th Floor
Boston, Massachusetts 02116
(617) 223-2312

U.S. Small Business Administration
150 Causeway Street, 10th Floor
Boston, Massachusetts 02114
(617) 223-3224

U.S. Small Business Administration
1550 Main Street
Springfield, Massachusetts 01103
(413) 785-0268

Associated Industries of
Massachusetts
462 Boylston Street
Boston, Massachusetts 02116
(617) 262-1180

Brockton Regional Chamber of
Commerce
One Centre Street
Brockton, Massachusetts 02401
(617) 586-0500

Central Berkshire Chamber of
Commerce
Berkshire Common
Pittsfield, Massachusetts 01201
(413) 499-4000

Chamber of Commerce of the
Attleboro Area
42 Union Street
Attleboro, Massachusetts 02703
(617) 222-0801

Fall River Area Chamber of
Commerce
P.O. Box 1871
200 Pocasset Street
Fall River, Massachusetts 02722
(617) 676-8226

Greater Boston Chamber of
Commerce
125 High Street
Boston, Massachusetts 02110
(617) 426-1250

Greater Fitchburg Chamber of
Commerce
344 Main Street
Fitchburg, Massachusetts 01420
(617) 343-6487

Greater Gardner Chamber of
Commerce
301 Central Street
Gardner, Massachusetts 01440

Greater Lawrence Chamber of
Commerce
300 Essex Street
Lawrence, Massachusetts 01840
(617) 687-9404

Greater Springfield Chamber of
Commerce
600 Bay State West Plaza, Suite 600
1500 Main Street
Springfield, Massachusetts 01115
(413) 734-5671

Massachusetts Department of
Commerce & Development
100 Cambridge Street
Boston, Massachusetts 02202
(617) 727-3218

Massachusetts Department of Food
& Agriculture
100 Cambridge Street
Boston, Massachusetts 02202
(617) 727-3108

New Bedford Area Chamber of
Commerce
Room 407,
First National Bank Building
New Bedford, Massachusetts 02742
(617) 999-5231

North Suburban Chamber of
Commerce
25-B Montvale Avenue
Woburn, Massachusetts 01801
(617) 933-3499

Office of Economic Affairs
One Ashburton Place
Boston, Massachusetts 02108
(617) 367-1830

South Middlesex Area Chamber of
Commerce
615 Concord Street
Framingham, Massachusetts 01701
(617) 879-5600

South Shore Chamber of Commerce
36 Miller Stile Road
Quincy, Massachusetts 02169
(617) 479-1111

Waltham/West Suburban Chamber
of Commerce
663 Main Street
Waltham, Massachusetts 02154
(617) 894-4700

Watertown Chamber of
Commerce
75 Main Street
Watertown, Massachusetts 02172
(617) 926-1017

Worcester Chamber of Commerce
Suite 350—Mechanics Tower
100 Front Street
Worcester, Massachusetts 01608
(617) 753-2924

Michigan

U.S. Department of Commerce
US & FCS District Office
445 Federal Building
231 West Lafayette
Detroit, Michigan 48226
(313) 226-3650

U.S. Small Business Administration
15 Patrick V. McNamara Building
477 Michigan Avenue, Room 515
Detroit, Michigan 48226
(313) 226-6075

U.S. Small Business Administration
220 W. Washington Street, Room 310
Marquette, Michigan 49885
(906) 225-1108

Ann Arbor Chamber of Commerce
207 East Washington
Ann Arbor, Michigan 48104
(313) 665-4433

City of Detroit
Community & Economic
Development Department
150 Michigan Avenue, 7th Floor
Detroit, Michigan 48226
(313) 224-6533

Detroit Customhouse Brokers &
Foreign Freight Forwarders
Association
1237-45 First National Building
Detroit, Michigan 48226
(313) 961-4130

Downriver Community Conference
15100 Northline
Southgate, Michigan 48195
(313) 283-8933

Flint Area Chamber of Commerce
708 Root
Flint, Michigan 49503
(313) 232-7101

(Greater) Detroit Chamber of
Commerce
150 Michigan Avenue

Detroit, Michigan 48226
(313) 964-4000

(Greater) Grand Rapids Chamber of
Commerce
17 Fountain Street, N.W.
Grand Rapids, Michigan 49502
(616) 459-7221

(Greater) Port Huron-Marysville
Chamber of Commerce
920 Pine Grove Avenue
Port Huron, Michigan 48060
(313) 985-7101

(Greater) Saginaw Chamber of
Commerce
901 S. Washington
Saginaw, Michigan 48606
(517) 752-7161

Kalamazoo Chamber of Commerce
500 W. Crosstown Parkway
Kalamazoo, Michigan 49008
(616) 381-4000

Macomb County Chamber of
Commerce
10 North Avenue
P.O. Box 855
Mt. Clemens, Michigan 48043
(313) 463-1528

Michigan Department of Agriculture
P.O. Box 30017
Lansing, Michigan 48909
(517) 373-1054

Michigan Manufacturers
Association
124 East Kalamazoo
Lansing, Michigan 48933
(517) 372-5900

Michigan State Chamber of
Commerce
Small Business Programs
200 N. Washington Square, Suite 400
Lansing, Michigan 48933
(517) 371-2100

Muskegon Area Chamber of
Commerce
1065 Fourth Street
Muskegon, Michigan 49441
(616) 722-3751

Office of International Development
Michigan Department of Commerce
Law Building, 5th Floor
Lansing, Michigan 48909
(517) 373-6390

Twin Cities Area Chamber of
Commerce
777 Riverview Drive, Building V
Benton Harbor, Michigan 49022
(616) 925-0044

West Michigan World Trade Club
445 Sixth Street, NW.
Grand Rapids, Michigan 49504
(616) 451-7651

World Trade Club of Detroit
150 Michigan Avenue
Detroit, Michigan 48226
(313) 964-4000

Minnesota

U.S. Department of Commerce
US&FCS District Office
108 Federal Building
110 S. 4th Street
Minneapolis, Minnesota 55401
(612) 349-3338

U.S. Small Business Administration
100 North 6th Street, Suite 610
Minneapolis, Minnesota 55403
(612) 349-3550

Minnesota Export Finance Authority
90 W. Plato Boulevard
St. Paul, Minnesota 55107
(612) 297-4659

Minnesota World Trade Association
33 E. Wentworth Avenue, 101
West St. Paul, Minnesota 55118
(612) 457-1038

Minnesota Trade Office
90 W. Plato Boulevard
St. Paul, Minnesota 55107
(612) 297-4222

Mississippi

U.S. Department of Commerce
US & FCS District Office
300 Woodrow Wilson Boulevard,
Suite 328
Jackson, Mississippi 39213
(601) 960-4388

U.S. Small Business Administration
100 West Capitol Street, Suite 322
Jackson, Mississippi 39269
(601) 960-4378

U.S. Small Business Administration
111 Fred Haise Boulevard,
2nd Floor
Biloxi, Mississippi 39530
(601) 435-3676

International Trade Club of
Mississippi, Inc.
P.O. Box 16673

Jackson, Mississippi 39236
(601) 981-7906

Marketing Division
Mississippi Department of Economic
Development
P.O. Box 849
Jackson, Mississippi 39205
(601) 359-3444

Missouri

U.S. Department of Commerce
US&FCS District Office
120 South Central, Suite 400
St. Louis, Missouri 53105
(314) 425-3301

U.S. Department of Commerce
US&FCS District Office
601 E. 12th Street, Room 635
Kansas City, Missouri 64106
(816) 374-3142

U.S. Small Business Administration
818 Grande Avenue
Kansas City, Missouri 64106
(816) 374-3419

U.S. Small Business Administration
309 North Jefferson, Room 150
Springfield, Missouri 65803
(417) 864-7670

International Business Development
Department of Commerce &
Economic Development
P.O. Box 118
Jefferson City, Missouri 65102
(314) 751-4855

International Trade Club of Greater
Kansas City

920 Main Street, Suite 600
Kansas City, Missouri 64105
(816) 221-1460

Missouri Department of Agriculture
International Marketing Division
P.O. Box 630
Jefferson City, Missouri 65102
(314) 751-5611

Missouri District Export Council
120 S. Central, Suite 400
St. Louis, Missouri 63105
(314) 425-3302

World Trade Club of St. Louis, Inc.
111 North Taylor Avenue
Kirkwood, Missouri 63122
(314) 965-9940

Montana

U.S. Department of Commerce
US&FCS District Office
(See listing for Denver, Colorado)

U.S. Small Business Administration
301 South Park, Room 528
Helena, Montana 59626
(406) 449-5381

U.S. Small Business Administration
Post-of-Duty
2601 First Avenue North, Room 216
Billings, Montana 59101
(406) 657-6047

Governor's Office of Commerce &
Small Business Development
State Capitol
Helena, Montana 59620
(406) 444-3923

Nebraska

U.S. Department of Commerce
US&FCS District Office
Empire State Building, 1st Floor
300 South 19th Street
Omaha, Nebraska 68102
(402) 221-3664

U.S. Small Business Administration
Empire State Building
300 South 19th Street
Omaha, Nebraska 68102
(402) 221-4691

International Division
Nebraska Department of Economic
Development
P.O. Box 94666
301 Centennial Mall South
Lincoln, Nebraska 68509
(402) 471-3111

Midwest International Trade
Association
c/o NBC, 13th & O Streets
Lincoln, Nebraska 68108
(402) 472-4321

Omaha Chamber of Commerce
International Affairs
1301 Harney Street
Omaha, Nebraska 68102
(402) 346-5000

Nevada

U.S. Department of Commerce
US&FCS District Office
1755 East Plumb Lane, Room 152
Reno, Nevada 89502
(702) 784-5203

U.S. Small Business Administration
301 East Steward Street
Las Vegas, Nevada 89125
(702) 385-6611

U.S. Small Business Administration
50 South Virginia Street,
Room 238
Reno, Nevada 89505
(702) 784-5268

Commission on Economic
Development
600 East Williams, Suite 203
Carson City, Nevada 89710
(702) 885-4325

Department of Economic
Development
Capitol Complex
Carson City, Nevada 89701
(701) 885-4325

Economic Development Authority
of Western Nevada
P.O. Box 11710
Reno, Nevada 89510
(702) 322-4004

Latin Chamber of Commerce
P.O. Box 7534
Las Vegas, Nevada 89125-2534
(702) 835-7367

Nevada Development Authority
P.O. Box 11128
Las Vegas, Nevada 89111

Nevada District Export Council
P.O. Box 11007
Reno, Nevada 89520
(702) 784-3401

New Hampshire

U.S. Department of Commerce
US&FCS District Office
(See listing for Boston,
Massachusetts)

U.S. Small Business Administration
55 Pleasant Street, Room 211
Concord, New Hampshire 03301
(603) 244-4041

Foreign Trade & Commercial
Development
Department of Resources &
Economic Development
105 Loudon Road, Building 2
Concord, New Hampshire 03301
(603) 271-2591

New Jersey

U.S. Department of Commerce
US&FCS District Office
3131 Princeton Pike, 4-D, Ste. 211
Trenton, New Jersey 08648
(609) 989-2100

U.S. Small Business Administration
60 Park Place, 4th Floor
Newark, New Jersey 07102
(201) 645-2434

U.S. Small Business Administration
1800 East Davis Street, Room 110
Camden, New Jersey 08104
(609) 757-5183

Department of Commerce &
Economic Development
Division of International Trade

242

744 Broad Street, Room 1709
Newark, New Jersey 07102
(201) 648-3518

World Trade Association of New
Jersey
5 Commerce Street
Newark, New Jersey 07102
(201) 623-7070

New Mexico

U.S. Department of Commerce
US&FCS District Office
517 Gold, SW., Ste 4303
Albuquerque, New Mexico 87102
(505) 766-2386

Department of Development
International Trade Division
Bataan Memorial Building
Santa Fe, New Mexico 87503
(505) 827-6208

New Mexico Department of
Agriculture
P.O. Box 5600
Las Cruces, New Mexico 88003
(505) 646-4929

New Mexico Foreign Trade and
Investment Council
Mail Stop 150, Alvarado Square
Albuquerque, New Mexico 87158
(505) 848-4632

New Mexico Industry Development
Corporation
5301 Central Avenue, N.E., Suite 705
Albuquerque, New Mexico 87110
(505) 262-2247

New York

U.S. Department of Commerce
US&FCS District Office
1312 Federal Building
111 West Huron Street
Buffalo, New York 14202
(716) 846-4191

U.S. Department of Commerce
US&FCS District Office
Federal Office Building,
Room 3718
26 Federal Plaza, Foley Square
New York, New York 10278
(212) 264-0634

U.S. Small Business Administration
26 Federal Plaza, Room 3100
New York, New York 10278
(212) 264-4355

U.S. Small Business Administration
35 Pinelawn Road, Room 102E
Melville, New York 11747
(516) 454-0750

U.S. Small Business Administration
100 S. Clinton Street, Room 1071
Syracuse, New York 13260
(315) 423-5383

U.S. Small Business Administration
111 West Huron Street,
Room 1311
Buffalo, New York 14202
(716) 846-4301

U.S. Small Business Administration
333 East Water Street
Elimira, New York 14901
(607) 733-4686

U.S. Small Business Administration
445 Broadway, Room 2368
Albany, New York 12207
(518) 472-6300

U.S. Small Business Administration
100 State Street, Room 601
Rochester, New York 14614
(716) 263-6700

Albany-Colonie Regional Chamber
of Commerce
14 Corporate Woods Boulevard
Albany, New York 12211
(518) 434-1214

American Association of Exporters
and Importers
11 West 42nd Street
New York, New York 10036
(212) 944-2230

Buffalo Area Chamber of Commerce
Economic Development
107 Delaware Avenue
Buffalo, New York 14202
(716) 849-6677

Buffalo World Trade Association
146 Canterbury Square
Williamsville, New York 14221
(716) 634-8439

Foreign Credit Insurance Association
One World Trade Center, 9th Floor
New York, New York 10048
(212) 432-6300

International Business Council of the
Rochester Area Chamber of
Commerce
International Trade & Transportation
55 St. Paul Street

Rochester, New York 14604
(716) 451-2220

Long Island Association, Inc.
80 Hauppage Road
Commack, New York 11725
(516) 499-4400

Long Island Association, Inc.
World Trade Club
Legislative & Economic Affairs
80 Hauppage Road
Commack, New York 11725
(516) 499-4400

Mohawk Valley World Trade Council
P.O. Box 4126
Utica, New York 13540
(315) 797-9530, Ext. 319

National Association of Export
Companies
200 Madison Avenue
New York, New York 10016
(212) 561-2025

New York Chamber of Commerce &
Industry
200 Madison Avenue
New York, New York 10016
(212) 561-2028

New York State Department of
Commerce
International Division
230 Park Avenue
New York, New York 10169
(212) 309-0502

Rochester Area Chamber of
Commerce
World Trade Department
International Trade & Transportation

55 St. Paul Street
Rochester, New York 14604
(716) 454-2220

Tappan Zee International Trade
Association
1 Blue Hill Plaza
Pearl River, New York 10965
(914) 735-7040

U.S. Council of the International
Chamber of Commerce
1212 Avenue of the Americas
New York, New York 10036
(212) 354-4480

Westchester County Association, Inc.
World Trade Club of Westchester
235 Mamaroneck Avenue
White Plains, New York 10605
(914) 948-6444

World Commerce Association of
Central New York
1 MONY Plaza
Syracuse, New York 13202
(315) 470-1343

World Trade Club of New York, Inc.
200 Madison Avenue
New York, New York 10016
(212) 561-2028

World Trade Institute
1 World Trade Center
New York, New York 10048
(212) 466-4044

North Carolina

U.S. Department of Commerce
US&FCS District Office

203 Federal Building
324 West Market Street
P.O. Box 1950
Greensboro, North Carolina 27402
(919) 378-5345

U.S. Small Business Administration
230 South Tryon Street, Room 700
Charlotte, North Carolina 28202
(704) 371-6563

U.S. Small Business Administration
215 South Evans Street, Room 102E
Greenville, North Carolina 27834
(919) 752-3798

Department of Commerce
International Division
430 North Salisburg Street
Raleigh, North Carolina 27611
(919) 733-7193

North Carolina Department of
Agriculture
P.O. Box 27647
Raleigh, North Carolina 27611
(919) 733-7912

North Carolina World Trade
Association
AMF Marine International
P.O. Box 2690
High Point, North Carolina 27261
(919) 899-6621

North Dakota

U.S. Department of Commerce
US&FCS District Office
(See listing for Omaha, Nebraska)

U.S. Small Business Administration
657 2nd Avenue, North, Room 218

Fargo, North Dakota 58108
(701) 237-5771

North Dakota Economic
Development Commission
International Trade Division
1050 E. Interstate Avenue
Bismarck, North Dakota 58505
(701) 224-2810

Fargo Chamber of Commerce
321 N. 4th Street
Fargo, North Dakota 58108
(701) 237-5678

Ohio

U.S. Department of Commerce
US&FCS District Office
9504 Federal Building
550 Main Street
Cincinnati, Ohio 45202
(513) 684-2944

U.S. Department of Commerce
US&FCS District Office
666 Enclid Avenue, Room 600
Cleveland, Ohio 44114
(216) 522-4750

U.S. Small Business
Administration
1240 East 9th Street, Room 317
Cleveland, Ohio 44199
(216) 552-4180

U.S. Small Business
Administration
85 Marconi Boulevard
Columbus, Ohio 43215
(614) 469-6860

U.S. Small Business Administration
550 Main Street, Room 5028
Cincinnati, Ohio 45202
(513) 684-2814

Cleveland World Trade
Association
690 Huntington Building
Cleveland, Ohio 44115
(216) 621-3300

Columbus Area Chamber of
Commerce
Economic Development
37 N. High Street
Columbus, Ohio 43216
(614) 221-1321

Columbus Council on
World Affairs
57 Jefferson Street
Columbus, Ohio 43215
(614) 461-0632

Commerce & Industry Association
of Greater Elyria
Elyria, Ohio 44036
(216) 322-5438

Dayton Council on World Affairs
300 College Park
Dayton, Ohio 45469
(513) 229-2319

Dayton Development Council
1880 Kettering Tower
Dayton, Ohio 45423
(513) 226-8222

Department of Development
International Trade Division
30 East Broad Street

P.O. Box 1001
Columbus, Ohio 43216
(614) 466-5017

(Greater) Cincinnati Chamber of
Commerce
Export Development
120 West 5th Street
Cincinnati, Ohio 45202
(513) 579-3122

(Greater) Cincinnati World Trade
Club
120 W. 5th Street
Cincinnati, Ohio 45202
(513) 579-3122

International Business & Trade
Association of Akron Regional
Development Board
Akron, Ohio 44308
(216) 376-5550

North Central Ohio Trade Club
Chamber of Commerce
Mansfield, Ohio 44902
(419) 522-3211

Ohio Department of Agriculture
Ohio Department Building, Room 607
65 South Front Street
Columbus, Ohio 43215
(614) 466-8789

Ohio Foreign Commerce
Association, Inc.
26250 Euclid Avenue, Suite 333
Cleveland, Ohio 44132
(216) 696-7000

Toledo Area International Trade
Association

Toledo, Ohio 43604
(419) 243-8191

Oklahoma

U.S. Department of Commerce
US&FCS District Office
4024 Lincoln Boulevard
Oklahoma City, Oklahoma 73105
(405) 231-5302

U.S. Small Business Administration
200 NW. 5th Street, Suite 670
Oklahoma City, Oklahoma 73102
(405) 231-4301

Department of Economic
Development
International Trade Division
4024 N. Lincoln Boulevard
P.O. Box 53424
Oklahoma City, Oklahoma 73152
(405) 521-3501

(Metropolitan) Tulsa Chamber of
Commerce
Economic Development Division
616 South Boston Avenue
Tulsa, Oklahoma 74119
(918) 585-1201

Oklahoma City Chamber of
Commerce
Economic and Community
Development
One Santa Fe Plaza
Oklahoma City, Oklahoma 73102
(405) 278-8900

Oklahoma City International Trade
Association
c/o Ditch Witch International

P.O. Box 66
Perry, Oklahoma 73077
(405) 336-4402

Oklahoma District Export Council
4024 Lincoln Boulevard
Oklahoma City, Oklahoma 73105
(405) 231-5302

Oklahoma State Chamber of
Commerce
4020 Lincoln Boulevard
Oklahoma City, Oklahoma 73105
(405) 424-4003

Tulsa World Trade Association
1821 N. 106th East Avenue
Tulsa, Oklahoma 74116
(918) 836-0338

Oregon

U.S. Department of Commerce
US & FCS District Office
1220 S.W. 3rd Avenue, Room 618
Portland, Oregon 97204
(503) 221-3001

U.S. Small Business Administration
1220 S.W. 3rd Avenue, Room 676
Portland, Oregon 97204
(503) 221-5221

Department of Economic
Development
International Trade Division
921 S.W. Washington, Suite 425
Portland, Oregon 97205
(503) 229-5625 or (800) 452-7813

Eugene Area Chamber of Commerce
1401 Willamette
P.O. Box 1107

Eugene, Oregon 97440
(503) 484-1314

Institute for International Trade and
Commerce
Portland State University
1912 S.W. 6th Avenue, Room 260
Portland, Oregon 97207
(503) 229-3246

Oregon District Export Council
1220 S.W. 3rd Avenue, Room 618
Portland, Oregon 97209
(503) 292-9219

Western Wood Products Association
Yem Building
Portland, Oregon 97204
(503) 224-3930

Pennsylvania

U.S. Department of Commerce
US&FCS District Office
9448 Federal Building
600 Arch Street
Philadelphia, Pennsylvania 19106
(215) 597-2866

U.S. Department of Commerce
US&FCS District Office
2002 Federal Building
1000 Liberty Avenue
Pittsburgh, Pennsylvania 15222
(412) 644-2850

U.S. Small Business Administration
231 St. Asaphs Road, Suite 400
Philadelphia, Pennsylvania 19004
(215) 596-5889

U.S. Small Business Administration
Branch Office

100 Chestnut Street, Suite 309
Harrisburg, Pennsylvania 17101
(717) 782-3840

U.S. Small Business Administration
Branch Office
20 North Pennsylvania Avenue
Wilkes-Barre, Pennsylvania 18701
(717) 826-6497

U.S. Small Business Administration
District Office
960 Pennsylvania Avenue, 5th Floor
Pittsburgh, Pennsylvania 15222
(412) 644-2780

American Society of International
Executives, Inc.
Dublin Hall, Suite 419
Blue Bell, Pennsylvania 19422
(215) 643-3040

(City of) Philadelphia
Municipal Services Bldg., Room 1660
Philadelphia, Pennsylvania 19102
(215) 686-3647

Economic Development Council of
Northwestern Pennsylvania
1151 Oak Street
Pittston, Pennsylvania 18640
(717) 655-5581

Erie Manufacturers Association
P.O. Box 1779
Erie, Pennsylvania 16507
(814) 453-4454

(Greater) Pittsburgh Chamber of
Commerce
411 Seventh Avenue
Pittsburgh, Pennsylvania 15219
(412) 392-4500

International Trade Development
Association
Box 113
Furlong, Pennsylvania 18925
(215) 822-6993

Pennsylvania Department of
Agriculture
Bureau of Agricultural
Development
2301 North Cameron Street
Harrisburg, Pennsylvania 17110
(717) 783-8460

Pennsylvania Department of
Commerce
Bureau of Domestic & International
Commerce
408 South Office Building
Harrisburg, Pennsylvania 17120
(717) 787-6500

Philadelphia Export Network
3508 Market Street, Suite 100
Philadelphia, Pennsylvania 19104
(215) 898-4189

Reading Foreign Trade
Association
35 N. 6th Street
Reading, Pennsylvania 19603
(215) 320-2976

Smaller Manufacturers Council
339 Boulevard of the Allies
Pittsburgh, Pennsylvania 15222
(412) 391-1622

Southwestern Pennsylvania
Economic Development District
355 Fifth Avenue, Room 1411
Pittsburgh, Pennsylvania 15222
(412) 391-1240

Western Pennsylvania District
Export Council
1000 Liberty Avenue, Room 2002
Pittsburgh, Pennsylvania 15222
(412) 644-2850

Women's International Trade
Association
P.O. Box 40004
Continental Station
Philadelphia, Pennsylvania 19106
(215) 923-6900

World Trade Association of
Philadelphia, Inc.
820 Land Title Building
Philadelphia, Pennsylvania 19110
(215) 563-8887

World Trade Club of Northwest
Pennsylvania
P.O. Box 1232
Kingston, Pennsylvania 18704
(717) 287-9624

Rhode Island

U.S. Department of Commerce
US&FCS District Office
(See listing for Boston,
Massachusetts)

U.S. Small Business
Administration
380 Westminster Mall
Providence, Rhode Island 02903
(401) 351-7500

Department of Economic
Development
7 Jackson Walkway

Providence, Rhode Island 02903
(401) 277-2601

South Carolina

U.S. Department of Commerce
US&FCS District Office
Strom Thurmond Federal Building,
Suite 172
1835 Assembly Street
Columbia, South Carolina 29201
(803) 765-5345

U.S. Small Business Administration
Strom Thurmond Federal Building,
Suite 172
1825 Assembly, 3rd Floor
Columbia, South Carolina 29202
(803) 765-5376

South Carolina District Export
Council
Strom Thurmond Federal Building,
Suite 172
1835 Assembly Street
Columbia, South Carolina 29201
(803) 765-5345

South Carolina International Trade
Club
Strom Thurmond Federal Building
Suite 172, 1835 Assembly Street
Columbia, South Carolina 29201
(803) 765-5345

South Carolina State Development
Board
International Division
P.O. Box 927
Columbia, South Carolina 29202
(803) 758-2235

South Dakota

U.S. Department of Commerce
US&FCS District Office
(See listing for Omaha, Nebraska)

U.S. Small Business Administration
101 South Main Avenue, Suite 101
Sioux Falls, South Dakota 57102
(605) 336-2980

Rapid City Area Chamber of
Commerce
P.O. Box 747
Rapid City, South Dakota 57709
(605) 343-1774

Sioux Falls Chamber of Commerce
127 E. 10th Street
Sioux Falls, South Dakota 57101
(605) 336-1620

South Dakota Bureau of Industrial
and Agricultural Development
221 S. Central
Pierre, South Dakota 57501
(605) 773-5032

Tennessee

U.S. Department of Commerce
US&FCS District Office
Suite 1114, Parkway Towers
404 James Robertson Parkway
Nashville, Tennessee 37219-1505
(615) 736-5161

U.S. Small Business Administration
404 James Robertson Parkway,
Suite 1012
Nashville, Tennessee 37219
(615) 251-5881

Chattanooga World Trade Council
1001 Market Street
Chattanooga, Tennessee 37402
(615) 765-2121

Department of Economic &
Community Development
Export Promotion Office
Andrew Jackson State Building,
Room 10
Nashville, Tennessee 37219
(615) 741-5870

East Tennessee International Trade
Club
c/o United American Bank
P.O. Box 280
Knoxville, Tennessee 37901
(615) 971-2027

Memphis World Trade Club
P.O. Box 3577
Memphis, Tennessee 38103
(901) 346-1001

Mid-South Exporters' Roundtable
P.O. Box 3521
Memphis, Tennessee 38103
(901) 761-3490

Middle Tennessee World Trade
Council
P.O. Box 17367
Nashville, Tennessee 37202
(615) 329-4931

Tennessee Department of
Agriculture
Ellington Agricultural Center
P.O. Box 40627, Melrose Station
Nashville, Tennessee 37204
(615) 360-0103

Tennessee District Export Council
c/o Aladdin Industries
P.O. Box 100255
Nashville, Tennessee 37210
(615) 748-3575

Texas

U.S. Department of Commerce
US&FCS District Office
1100 Commerce Street, Room 7A5
Dallas, Texas 75242
(214) 767-0542

U.S. Department of Commerce
US&FCS District Office
2625 Federal Building
515 Rusk Street
Houston, Texas 77002
(713) 229-2578

U.S. Small Business Administration
300 East 8th Street, Room 780
Austin, Texas 78701
(512) 482-5288

U.S. Small Business Administration
400 Mann Street, Suite 403
Corpus Christi, Texas 78408
(512) 888-3331

U.S. Small Business Administration
1100 Commerce Street, Room 3C36
Dallas, Texas 75242
(214) 767-0605

U.S. Small Business Administration
4100 Rio Bravo, Suite 300
El Paso, Texas 79902
(915) 543-7586

U.S. Small Business Administration
221 West Lancaster Avenue,

Room 1007
Ft. Worth, Texas 76102
(817) 334-5463

U.S. Small Business Administration
222 East Van Buren Street,
Room 500
Harlingen, Texas 78550
(512) 423-8934

U.S. Small Business Administration
2525 Murworth, Room 112
Houston, Texas 77054
(713) 660-4401

U.S. Small Business Administration
1611 Tenth Street, Suite 200
Lubbock, Texas 79401
(806) 762-7466

U.S. Small Business Administration
100 South Washington Street,
Room 3C36
Marshall, Texas 75670
(214) 935-5257

U.S. Small Business
Administration
727 East Duranyo Street,
Room A-513
San Antonio, Texas 78206
(512) 229-6250

Amarillo Chamber of Commerce
Amarillo Building
1301 S. Polk
Amarillo, Texas 79101
(806) 374-5238

Dallas Chamber of Commerce
1507 Pacific
Dallas, Texas 75201
(214) 954-1111

Dallas Council on World Affairs
The Fred Lange Center
1310 Annex, Suite 101
Dallas, Texas 75204
(214) 827-7960

El Paso Chamber of Commerce
10 Civic Center Plaza
El Paso, Texas 79944
(915) 544-7880

Foreign Credit Insurance Association
600 Travis
Suite 2860
Houston, Texas 77002
(713) 227-0987

Fort Worth Chamber of Commerce
700 Throckmorton
Fort Worth, Texas 76102
(817) 336-2491

Greater San Antonio Chamber of
Commerce
P.O. Box 1628
San Antonio, Texas 78296
(512) 227-8181

Houston Chamber of Commerce
1100 Milam Building, 25th Floor
Houston, Texas 77002
(713) 651-1313

Houston World Trade Association
1520 Texas Avenue, Suite 239
Houston, Texas 77002
(713) 225-0967

Lubbock Chamber of Commerce
14th Street & Avenue K
P.O. Box 561
Lubbock, Texas 79408
(806) 763-4666

North Texas Customs Brokers &
Foreign Freight Forwarders
Association
P.O. Box 225464
DFW Airport, Texas 75261
(214) 456-0730

Odessa Chamber of Commerce
P.O. Box 3626
Odessa, Texas 79760
(915) 322-9111

Texas Department of
Agriculture
Export Services Division
P.O. Box 12847, Capitol Station
Austin, Texas 78711
(512) 475-2760

Texas Economic Development
Commission
International Trade
Department
P.O. Box 13561
Austin, Texas 78711
(512) 475-6156

Texas Industrial Development
Council, Inc.
P.O. Box 1002
College Station, Texas 77841
(409) 845-2911

U.S. Chamber of Commerce
4835 LBJ Freeway, Suite 750
Dallas, Texas 75324
(214) 387-0404

World Trade Association of
Dallas/Fort Worth
P.O. Box 29334
Dallas, Texas 75229
(214) 760-9105

Utah

U.S. Department of Commerce
US&FCS District Office
U.S. Post Office Building, Room 340
350 South Main Street
Salt Lake City, Utah 84101
(801) 524-5116

U.S. Small Business Administration
125 South State Street, Room 2237
Salt Lake City, Utah 84138
(314) 524-5800

Salt Lake Area Chamber of
Commerce
Export Development Committee
19 E. 2nd Street
Salt Lake City, Utah 84111

Utah Economic & Industrial
Development Division
6150 State Office Building
Salt Lake City, Utah 84114
(801) 533-5325

World Trade Association of Utah
10 Exchange Place
Suite 301–302
Salt Lake City, Utah 84111
(801) 531-1515

Vermont

U.S. Department of Commerce
US & FCS District Office
(See listing for Boston,
Massachusetts)

U.S. Small Business Administration
87 State Street, Room 204
Montpelier, Vermont 05602
(802) 229-0538

Department of Economic
Development
Pavilion Office Building
Montpelier, Vermont 05602
(802) 828-3221

Virginia

U.S. Department of Commerce
US&FCS District Office
8010 Federal Building
400 North 8th Street
Richmond, Virginia 23240
(804) 771-2246

U.S. Small Business Administration
3015 Federal Building
400 North 8th Street
Richmond, Virginia 23240
(804) 771-2617

International Trade Association of
Northern Virginia
P.O. Box 2982
Reston, Virginia 22090

International Trade Development
Division of Industrial
Development
1010 Washington Building
Richmond, Virginia 23219
(804) 786-3791

Newport News Export Trading
System
Department of Development
Peninsula Export Program
2400 Washington Avenue
Newport News, Virginia 32607
(804) 247-8751

Piedmont Foreign Trade Council
P.O. Box 1374

Lynchburg, Virginia 24505
(804) 782-4231

Vextrac/Export Trading Company of
the Virginia Port Authority
600 World Trade Center
Norfolk, Virginia 23510
(804) 623-8000

(Virginia) Chamber of Commerce
611 E. Franklin Street
Richmond, Virginia 23219
(804) 644-1607

Virginia Department of Agriculture
& Consumer Services
1100 Bank Street, Room 710
Richmond, Virginia 23219
(804) 786-3501

Virginia District Export Council
P.O. Box 10190
Richmond, Virginia 23240
(804) 771-2246

Washington

U.S. Department of Commerce
706 Lake Union Building
1700 Westlake Avenue North
Seattle, Washington 98109
(206) 442-5616

U.S. Small Business Administration
915 Second Avenue, Room 1792
Seattle, Washington 98174
(206) 442-5534

U.S. Small Business Administration
W920 Riverside Avenue, Room 651
Spokane, Washington 99210
(509) 456-5310

Department of Commerce &
Economic Development
International Trade & Investment
Division
312 1st Avenue North
Seattle, Washington 89109
(206) 348-7149

Economic Development Council of
Puget Sound
1218 Third Avenue, Suite 1900
Seattle, Washington 98101
(206) 622-2868

Inland Empire World Trade Club
P.O. Box 3727
Spokane, Washington 99220
(509) 489-0500

Seattle Chamber of Commerce Trade
& Transportation Division
One Union Square, 12th Floor
Seattle, Washington 98101
(206) 447-7263

Washington Council on International
Trade
Suite 420
Fourth and Vine Building
Seattle, Washington 98121
(206) 621-8485

Washington State Department of
Agriculture
406 General Administration Building
Olympia, Washington 98504
(206) 753-5046

Washington State International Trade
Fair
312 First Avenue North
Seattle, Washington 98109
(206) 682-6911

World Affairs Council
Mayflower Park Hotel
405 Olive Way
Seattle, Washington 98101
(206) 682-6986

World Trade Club of Bellevue
100 116th Avenue S.E.
Bellevue, Washington 98005
(206) 454-2464

World Trade Club of Seattle
1402 Third Avenue, Suite 414
Seattle, Washington 98101
(206) 621-0344

West Virginia

U.S. Department of Commerce
US & FCS District Office
3000 New Federal Office
Building
500 Quarrier Street
Charleston, West Virginia 25301
(304) 347-5123

U.S. Small Business
Administration
168 West Main Street
Clarksburg, West Virginia 26301
(304) 923-3706

U.S. Small Business
Administration
628 Charleston National Plaza
Charleston, West Virginia 25301
(304) 347-5220

Governor's Office of Economic &
Community Development
State Capitol, Room B-517
Charleston, West Virginia 25305
(304) 348-2234

West Virginia Chamber of
Commerce
P.O. Box 2789
Charleston, West Virginia 25330
(304) 342-1115

West Virginia District Export
Council
P.O. Box 26
Charleston, West Virginia 25321
(304) 343-8874

West Virginia Manufacturers
Association
1313 Charleston National Plaza
Charleston, West Virginia 25301
(304) 342-2123

Wisconsin

U.S. Department of Commerce
US&FCS District Office
605 Federal Building
517 East Wisconsin Avenue
Milwaukee, Wisconsin 53202
(414) 291-3473

U.S. Small Business Administration
212 East Washington Avenue,
Room 213
Madison, Wisconsin 53703
(608) 264-5261

U.S. Small Business Administration
500 South Barstow Street, Room 17
Eau Claire, Wisconsin 54701
(715) 834-9012

U.S. Small Business Administration
310 West Wisconsin Avenue,
Room 400
Milwaukee, Wisconsin 53203
(414) 291-3941

Milwaukee Association of
Commerce
756 N. Milwaukee Street
Milwaukee, Wisconsin 53202
(414) 273-3000

Small Business Development
Center
602 State Street
Madison, Wisconsin 53703
(608) 263-7766

Wisconsin Department of
Development
123 West Washington Avenue
Madison, Wisconsin 53702
(608) 266-1767

Wyoming

U.S. Department of Commerce
US&FCS District Office
(See listing for Denver, Colorado)

U.S. Small Business Administration
100 East "B" Street, Room 4001
Casper, Wyoming 82602
(307) 261-5761

Wyoming Department of Commerce
International Trade Office
Herschler Building 2W
122 West 25th Street
Cheyenne, Wyoming 82002
(307) 777-2412

Appendix 2
International Trade
Administration/US&FCS District Offices

Alabama

Rm. 302
2015 2nd Ave. North
Berry Bldg.
Birmingham, Alabama 35203
(205) 731-1331

Alaska

701 C St.
P.O. Box 32
Anchorage, Alaska 99513
(907) 271-5041

Arizona

Federal Bldg. & U.S. Courthouse
230 North 1st Ave.

Rm. 3412
Phoenix, Arizona 85025
(602) 261-3285

Arkansas

Suite 811
Savers Fed. Bldg.
320 W. Capitol Ave.
Little Rock, Arkansas 72201
(501) 378-5794

California

Rm. 800
11777 San Vicente Blvd.
Los Angeles, California 90049
(213) 209-6707

116-A W. 4th St.
Suite #1
Santa Ana, California 92701
(714) 836-2461

6363 Greenwich Dr.
San Diego, California 92122
(619) 557-5395

Fed. Bldg.
Box 36013
450 Golden Gate Ave.
San Francisco, California 94102
(415) 556-5860

Colorado

Rm. 119
U.S. Customhouse
721-19th St.
Denver, Colorado 80202
(303) 844-3246

Connecticut

Rm. 610-B
Fed. Office Bldg.
450 Main St.
Hartford, Connecticut 06103
(203) 240-3530

Delaware

Serviced by Philadelphia District
Office

District of Columbia

(Baltimore, Md. District)
Rm. 1066 HCHB
Department of Commerce

14th St. & Constitution Ave.,
N.W.
Washington, D.C. 20230
(202) 377-3181

Florida

Suite 224
Fed. Bldg.
51 S.W. First Ave.
Miami, Florida 33130
(305) 536-5267

128 North Osceola Ave.
Clearwater, Florida 33515
(813) 461-0011

3100 University Blvd. South
Jacksonville, Florida 32216
(904) 791-2796

75 East Ivanhoe Blvd.
Orlando, Florida 32804
(305) 425-1234

Collins Bldg.
Rm. 401
107 W. Gaines St.
Tallahassee, Florida 32304
(904) 488-6469

Georgia

Suite 504
1365 Peachtree St., N.E.
Atlanta, Georgia 30309
(404) 347-4872

120 Barnard St.
A-107
Savannah, Georgia 31402
(912) 944-4204

Hawaii

4106 Fed. Bldg.
P.O. Box 50026
300 Ala Moana Blvd.
Honolulu, Hawaii 96850
(808) 541-1782

Idaho

(Denver, Colorado District)
Statehouse, Room 113
Boise, Idaho 83720
(208) 334-9254

Illinois

1406 Mid Continental Plaza Bldg.
55 East Monroe St.
Chicago, Illinois 60603
(312) 353-4450

W.R. Harper College
Algonquin & Roselle Rd.
Palatine, Illinois 60067
(312) 397-3000, x-532

515 North Court St.
P.O. Box 1747
Rockford, Illinois
61110-0247
(815) 987-8100

Indiana

357 U.S. Courthouse & Fed.
Office Bldg.
46 East Ohio St.
Indianapolis, Indiana 46204
(317) 269-6214

Iowa

817 Fed. Bldg.
210 Walnut St.
Des Moines, 50309
(515) 284-4222

Kansas

(Kansas City, Missouri District)
River Park Pl., Suite 565
727 North Waco
Wichita, Kansas 67203
(316) 269-6160

Kentucky

Rm. 636B
U.S. Post Office and Courthouse
Bldg.
Louisville, Kentucky 40202
(502) 582-5066

Louisiana

432 World Trade Center,
No. 2 Canal St.
New Orleans, Louisiana 70130
(504) 589-6546

Maine

(Boston, Massachusetts
District)
1 Memorial Circle
Casco Bank Bldg.
Augusta, Maine 04330
(207) 622-8249

Maryland

415 U.S. Customhouse
Gay and Lombard Sts.
Baltimore, Maryland 21202
(301) 962-3560

Massachusetts

World Trade Center
Suite 307
Commonwealth Pier Area
Boston, Massachusetts 02210
(617) 565-8563

Michigan

1140 McNamara Bldg.
477 Michigan Ave.
Detroit, Michigan 48226
(313) 226-3650

300 Monroe N.W.
Rm. 409
Grand Rapids, Michigan 49503
(616) 456-2411

Minnesota

108 Fed. Bldg.
110 S. 4th St.
Minneapolis, Minnesota 55401
(612) 348-1638

Mississippi

328 Jackson Mall Office Center
300 Woodrow Wilson Blvd.
Jackson, Mississippi 39213
(601) 965-4388

Missouri

7911 Forsyth Blvd.
Suite 610
St. Louis, Missouri 63105
(314) 425-3302-4

Rm. 635
601 East 12th St.
Kansas City, Missouri 64106
(816) 426-3141

Montana

Serviced by Denver District
Office

Nebraska

11133 "O" St.
Omaha, Nebraska 68137
(402) 221-3664

Nevada

1755 E. Plumb Ln., #152
Reno, Nevada 89502
(702) 784-5203

New Hampshire

Serviced by Boston District
Office

New Jersey

3131 Princeton Pike Bldg. 6
Suite 100
Trenton, New Jersey 08648
(609) 989-2100

New Mexico

517 Gold, S.W.
Suite 4303
Albuquerque, New Mexico 87102
(505) 766-2386

New York

1312 Fed. Bldg.
111 West Huron St.
Buffalo, New York 14202
(716) 846-4191

121 East Ave.
Rochester, New York 14604
(716) 263-6480

Fed. Office Bldg.
26 Fed. Plaza
Rm. 3718, Foley Sq.
New York, New York 10278
(212) 264-0634

North Carolina

324 W. Market St.
P.O. Box 1950
Greensboro, North Carolina 27402
(919) 333-5345

North Dakota

Serviced by Omaha District Office

Ohio

9504 Fed. Office Bldg.
550 Main St.
Cincinnati, Ohio 45202
(513) 684-2944

Rm. 600
666 Euclid Ave.
Cleveland, Ohio 44114
(216) 522-4750

Oklahoma

5 Broadway Executive Park, Suite 200
6601 Broadway Extension
Oklahoma City, Oklahoma 73116
(405) 231-5302

440 S. Houston St.
Tulsa, Oklahoma 74127
(918) 581-7650

Oregon

Rm. 618
1220 S.W. 3rd Ave.
Portland, Oregon 97204
(503) 221-3001

Pennsylvania

9448 Fed. Bldg.
600 Arch St.
Philadelphia, Pennsylvania 19106
(215) 597-2866

2002 Fed. Bldg.
1000 Liberty Ave.
Pittsburgh, Pennsylvania 15222
(412) 644-2850

Puerto Rico

Rm. 659-Fed. Bldg.
San Juan (Hato Rey),
Puerto Rico 00918
(809) 753-4555

Rhode Island

(Boston, Massachusetts District)
7 Jackson Walkway
Providence, Rhode Island 02903
(401) 528-5104, ext. 22

South Carolina

Strom Thurmond Fed. Bldg.
Suite 172
1835 Assembly St.
Columbia, South Carolina 29201
(803) 765-5345

17 Lockwood Dr.
Charleston, South Carolina 29401
(803) 724-4361

South Dakota

Serviced by Omaha District
Office

Tennessee

Suite 1114
Parkway Towers
404 James Robertson Parkway
Nashville, Tennessee 37219-1505
(615) 736-5161

555 Beale St.
Memphis, Tennessee 38103
(901) 521-4137

Texas

Rm. 7A5, 1100 Commerce St.
Dallas, Texas 75242
(214) 767-0542

P.O. Box 12728
Capitol Station
Austin, Texas 78711
(512) 472-5059

2625 Fed. Courthouse
515 Rusk St.
Houston, Texas 77002
(713) 229-2578

Utah

Rm. 340 U.S. Courthouse
350 S. Main St.
Salt Lake City, Utah 84101
(801) 524-5116

Vermont

Serviced by Boston District
Office

Virginia

8010 Fed. Bldg.
400 North 8th St.
Richmond, Virginia 23240
(804) 771-2246

Washington

3131 Elliott Ave.
Suite 290
Seattle, Washington 98121
(206) 442-5616

P.O. Box 2170
Spokane, Washington 99210
(509) 456-4557

West Virginia

3309 Fed. Bldg.
500 Quarrier St.
Charleston, West Virginia 25301
(304) 347-5123

Wisconsin

Fed. Bldg., U.S. Courthouse
517 E. Wisc. Ave.

Milwaukee, Wisconsin 53202
(414) 291-3473

Wyoming

Serviced by Denver District
Office

The Federal Government

Small Business Administration (SBA)

Background

The SBA offers the small business owner a variety of direct services. It also serves as the advocate for small business within the federal government.

Counseling is provided for the business owner or potential business owner, especially in the start-up phases, including business plans and other subjects necessary to launch a business. The assistance can take the form of individual counseling or prebusiness workshops. The SBA also offers numerous publications on all facets of small business matters.

Most dealings with the SBA are best handled at the district or regional office level. For this reason, a directory of those offices has been included in this section. If you still have questions after contacting the office closest to you, telephone numbers at the national level have been included according to the programs they oversee.

1441 L St., NW, Washington, DC 20416
(800) 368-5855
(202) 653-7561

Financial Assistance (202) 653-6470

The SBA provides guaranteed, direct, or immediate participation loans to small business concerns to help them finance plant construction, conversion, or expansion. The loans can also be used to acquire equipment, facilities, and supplies. It should be noted that direct loan funds are limited; most assistance is provided through SBA guarantees of loans provided by local banks. Catastrophe victims are provided with loans to aid them in rebuilding or replacing their businesses. Handicapped individuals and their employers may also be eligible for certain assistance.

The following programs or services are offered in this area:

- Contract loans
- Disaster assistance to non agricultural businesses
- Economic injury
- Export revolving line of credit
- Handicapped assistance loans
- Physical disaster loans
- Small business investment companies

- Regular business loans
- Seasonal line of credit
- Energy loans
- Disaster loans
- Economic opportunity loans
- Loan development companies
- Pollution control loans
- Section 503 certified development company assistance

Procurement Assistance (202) 653-6508

The SBA provides a wide range of services to help small businesses obtain and fulfill government contracts. Through set-asides for small businesses, subcontracting opportunities with larger companies, and a computerized small business source referral system, the SBA works to increase the number of contracts going to small business. It also has procurement center representatives stationed at all federal installations, both military and civilian, that have major buying programs. They help review procurement packages and provide counseling.

The following programs or services are offered in this area:

- Prime contracts: referrals and information
- Procurement automated source systems
- Property sales
- Surety bond guarantees
- Labor surplus area set-asides
- Subcontracting
- Certificate of competency

Business Development (202) 653-6330

Assistance is available from the SBA for existing and prospective small businesses in several forms with the objectives of improving their management and operational skills. This office can advise small businesses about programs and services offered within the SBA and other federal departments and agencies. Types of assistance available include, but are not limited to:

- Workshops for prospective business owners
- Management counseling, including SCORE (Service Corps of Retired Executives), ACE (Active Corps of Executives), graduate and undergraduate students of business management schools participating in the Small Business Institute Program, and other volunteer groups
- Management courses, conferences, and clinics
- Publications to assist in management of small business
- Small Business Development Centers (SBDCs) offer extensive university-based counseling and training programs.

Through a cooperative arrangement between the SBA and the Veterans Administration, special business ownership training is available to eligible veterans. Special publications and counseling on technology in the management and operations field are also available. There are two publications available from the SBA that list all the publications that are available:

- Business Development Pamphlet 115A
- Business Development Booklet 115B

The following programs or services are offered in this area:

- Small business development centers
- Small business institutes
- Professional and technical assistance
- Specialized subject matter workshops
- Prebusiness workshops
- Publications
- SCORE/ACE

Advocacy (202) 653-6808

The Office of Advocacy represents the interests of small businesses before the federal government. The Office of Interagency Affairs analyzes proposed laws and regulations to determine potential impact on small businesses and provides advice and counsel to Federal agencies on ways to minimize adverse effects or to maximize benefits in particular situations. The Office of Economic Research maintains extensive databases on small business and conducts research on economic policy issues important to small business. The Office of Information publishes directories and pamphlets, and issues summaries on legislative and regulatory issues.

The following programs or services are offered in this area:

- Small business data base development
- Information: directories, issue papers, economic data
- Small business economic research
- Ombudsman services
- Regulatory flexibility monitoring

Minority Business Development (MBD) (202) 653-5688

The main objective of MBD is to help close the gap in business ownership between minority individuals and those in the majority. The SBA has combined its efforts with those of private industry, banks, local communities, and other government agencies to meet those goals.

The following programs or services are offered in this area:

- Call contracts for technical assistance
- Call contracts
- 8(a) certification procurement contract
- Minority enterprise small business investment companies (MESBICS)

International Trade Assistance (ITA) (202) 653-7794

The ITA offers many of the programs found elsewhere within the SBA. The programs are targeted toward businesses which specialize in the area of international trade and range from technical and managerial assistance to financial assistance.

SBA Field Offices

Following is a listing of the addresses and telephone numbers of SBA field offices around the country. Most of the programs and services of the SBA are administered and delivered through these field offices.

Several types of offices are listed and they are categorized by region. The first office listed in each region is the regional office. The others are district or branch offices. To begin communication with the SBA, contact the office nearest you and ascertain what programs and services it offers. If it does not have what you are looking for, it will refer you to the nearest office which does.

Region I

Boston 60 Batterymarch Street, 10th Floor, Boston, Massachusetts 02110 (617) 223-3204
Boston 150 Causeway St., 10th Floor, Boston, Massachusetts 02114 (617) 223-3224

Springfield   1550 Main Street, Springfield, Massachusetts 01108 (413) 785-0268
Augusta   40 Western Ave., Room 512, Augusta, Maine 04330 (207) 622-8378
Concord   Post Office Building, 55 Pleasant St., Room 209, Concord, New Hampshire 03301 (603) 224-4041
Hartford   One Hartford Square West, Hartford, Connecticut 06106 (203) 722-3600
Montpelier   87 State St., Room 204, Montpelier, Vermont 05602 (802) 229-0538
Providence   380 Westminster Mall, Providence, Rhode Island 02903 (401) 528-4561

Region II

New York   26 Federal Plaza, Room 29-118, New York, New York 10278 (212) 264-7772
New York   26 Federal Plaza, Room 3100, New York, New York 10278 (212) 264-4355
Melville   35 Pinelawn Road, Room 102E, Melville, New York 11747 (516) 454-0750
Hato Rey   Federal Building, Carlos Chardon Ave., Room 691, Hato Rey, Puerto Rico 00918 (809) 753-4002
St. Croix   United Shopping Center, Suite 7, Cristiensted, St. Croix, Virgin Islands 00820 (809) 773-3480
St. Thomas   Veterans Drive, Room 283, St. Thomas, Virgin Islands 00801 (809) 774-8530
Newark   60 Park Place, 4th Floor, Newark, New Jersey 07102 (201) 645-2434
Camden   1800 E. Davis St., Room 110, Camden, New Jersey 08104 (609) 757-5183
Syracuse   100 S. Clinton St., Room 1071, Syracuse, New York 13260 (315) 423-5383
Buffalo   111 W. Huron St., Room 1311, Buffalo, New York 14202 (716) 846-4301
Elmira   333 E. Water St., Elmira, New York 14901 (607) 734-8130

Albany   445 Broadway, Room 236B, Albany, New York 12207 (518) 472-6300
Rochester   100 State St., Rochester, New York 14614 (716) 263-6700

Region III

Philadelphia   1 Bala Plaza, Suite 640, Bala-Cynwyd, Pennsylvania 19004 (215) 596-5889
Philadelphia   1 Bala Plaza, Suite 400, Bala-Cynwyd, Pennsylvania 19004 (215) 596-5889
Harrisburg   100 Chestnut St., Suite 309, Harrisburg, Pennsylvania 17101 (717) 782-3840
Wilkes-Barre   20 N. Pennsylvania Ave., Room 2327, Wilkes-Barre, Pennsylvania 18701 (717) 826-6497
Wilmington   844 King St., Room 5207, Wilmington, Delaware 19801 (302) 573-6294
Clarksburg   168 W. Main St., Room 302, Clarksburg, West Virginia 26301 (304) 623-5631
Charleston   550 Eagan St., Charleston, West Virginia 25301 (304) 347-5220
Pittsburgh   960 Penn Ave., 5th Floor, Pittsburgh, Pennsylvania 15222 (412) 644-2780
Richmond   400 North 8th St., Room 3015, Richmond, Virginia 23240 (804) 771-2617
Baltimore   10 N. Calvert St., Baltimore, Maryland 21202 (301) 962-4392
Washington   1111 18th St., NW, 6th Floor, Washington, DC 20036 (202) 634-4950

Region IV

Atlanta   1375 Peachtree St., N.E., Suite 502, Atlanta, Georgia 30367 (404) 881-4999
Atlanta   1720 Peachtree Rd., N.W., 6th Floor, Atlanta, Georgia 30309 (404) 881-4749

Statesboro   Federal Building, 52 N. Main St., Room 225, Statesboro, Georgia 30458 (912) 489-8719

Birmingham   2121 8th Ave. North, Suite 200, Birmingham, Alabama 35203-2398 (205) 254-1344

Charlotte   230 S. Tryon St., Room 700, Charlotte, North Carolina 28202 (704) 371-6563

Columbia   1835 Assembly St., 3rd Floor, Columbia, South Carolina 29202 (803) 765-5376

Jackson   100 W. Capitol St., Suite 322, Jackson, Mississippi 39269 (601) 960-4378

Gulfport   1 Hancock Plaza, Suite 1001, Gulfport, Mississippi 39501 (601) 863-4449

Jacksonville   400 W. Bay St., Room 261, Jacksonville, Florida 32202 (904) 791-3782

Louisville   600 Federal Place, Room 188, Louisville, Kentucky 40201 (502) 582-5971

Coral Gables   2222 Ponce De Leon Blvd., 5th Floor, Coral Gables, Florida 33134 (305) 536-5521

Tampa   700 Twiggs St., Room 607, Tampa, Florida 33602 (813) 228-2594

West Palm Beach   3500 45th St., Suite 6, West Palm Beach, Florida 33407 (305) 689-2223

Nashville   404 James Robertson Parkway, Suite 1012, Nashville Tennessee 37219 (615) 251-5881

Region V

Chicago   230 S. Dearborn St., Room 510, Chicago, Illinois 60604 (312) 353-0359

Chicago   219 S. Dearborn St., Room 437, Chicago, Illinois 60604 (312) 353-4528

Cleveland   Federal Building, 1240 East 9th St., Room 317, Cleveland, Ohio 44199 (216) 522-4180

Columbus   85 Marconi Blvd., Columbus, Ohio 43215 (619) 469-6860

Cincinnati   550 Main St., Room 5028, Cincinnati, Ohio 45202 (513) 684-2814

Detroit   Patrick McNamara Bldg., 477 Michigan Ave., Room
515, Detroit, Michigan 48226 (313) 226-6075
Marquette   220 W. Washington St., Room 310, Marquette,
Michigan 49855 (906) 225-1108
Indianapolis   575 N. Pennsylvania St., Room 578, Indianapolis,
Indiana 46204 (317) 269-7272
Madison   212 E. Washington Ave., Room 213, Madison, Wis-
consin 53703 (608) 264-5261
Eau Claire   500 S. Barstow St., Room 17, Eau Claire, Wisconsin
54701 (715) 834-9012
Milwaukee   310 W. Wisconsin Ave., Room 400, Milwaukee,
Wisconsin 53203 (414) 291-3941
Minneapolis   Butler Square, 100 North 6th St., Suite 610, Min-
neapolis, Minnesota 55403 (612) 349-3550
Springfield   Four North, Old State Capital Plaza, Springfield,
Illinois 62701 (217) 492-4416

Region VI

Dallas   8625 King George Dr., Bldg. C., Dallas, Texas 75235
(214) 767-7643
Dallas   1100 Commerce St., Room 3C36, Dallas, Texas 75242
(214) 767-0605
Marshall   505 E. Travis Terrace Bldg., Room 103, Marshall,
Texas 75670 (214) 935-5257
El Paso   10737 Gateway West, Suite 320, El Paso, Texas 79935
(915) 541-7678
Ft. Worth   819 Taylor St., 10A27, Ft. Worth, Texas 76102 (817)
334-3777
Albuquerque   5000 Marble Ave., N.E., Room 320, Albuquer-
que, New Mexico 87100 (505) 766-3430
Harlingen   222 E. Van Buren St., Room 500, Harlingen, Texas
78550 (512) 423-8934
Corpus Christi   400 Mann St., Suite 403, Corpus Christi, Texas
78401 (512) 888-3331
Houston   2525 Murworth, Room 112, Houston, Texas 77054
(713) 660-4401

Little Rock   320 W. Capitol Ave., Room 601, Little Rock, Arkansas 72201 (501) 378-5871

Lubbock   1611 Tenth St., Suite 200, Lubbock, Texas 79401 (806) 743-7466

New Orleans   1661 Canal St., Suite 2000, New Orleans, Louisiana 70112 (504) 589-6685

Shreveport   500 Fannin St., Room 6B14, Shreveport, Louisiana 71101 (318) 226-5196

Oklahoma City   200 N.W. 5th St., Suite 670, Oklahoma City, Oklahoma 73102 (405) 231-4301

San Antonio   727 E. Durango Blvd., Room A-513, San Antonio, Texas 78206 (512) 229-6250

Austin   300 East 8th St., Room 520, Austin, Texas 78701 (512) 482-5288

Region VII

Kansas City   911 Walnut St., 13th Floor, Kansas City, Missouri 64106 (816) 374-5288

Kansas City   1103 Grande Ave., Kansas City, Missouri 64106 (816) 374-3419

Springfield   309 N. Jefferson, Suite 150, Springfield, Missouri 65805 (417) 864-7670

Cedar Rapids   373 Collins Rd. N.E., Cedar Rapids, Iowa 52402 (319) 399-2571

Des Moines   210 Walnut St., Room 749, Des Moines, Iowa 50309 (515) 284-4422

Omaha   300 South 19th St., Omaha, Nebraska 68102 (402) 221-4691

St. Louis   815 Olive St., Room 242, St. Louis, Missouri 63101 (314) 425-6600

Cape Girardeau   101 W. Main, Cape Girardeau, Missouri 63755 (314) 335-6039

Wichita   110 E. Waterman St., Wichita, Kansas 67202 (316) 269-6571

Region VIII

Denver   1405 Curtis St., 22nd Floor, Denver, Colorado 80202 (303) 844-5441

Denver   721 19th St., Room 407, Denver, Colorado 80202 (303) 844-2607

Casper   100 East B Street, Room 4001, Casper, Wyoming 82601 (307) 261-5761

Fargo   657 2nd Ave., North, Room 218, Fargo, North Dakota 58102 (701) 237-5771

Helena   301 S. Park, Room 528, Helena, Montana 59626 (406) 449-5381

Billings   2601 First Ave. North, Room 216, Billings, Montana 59101 (406) 657-6047

Salt Lake City   125 S. State St., Room 2237, Salt Lake City, Utah 84138 (801) 524-5800

Sioux Falls   101 S. Main Ave., Suite 101, Sioux Falls, South Dakota 57102 (605) 336-2980

Region IX

San Francisco   450 Golden Gate Ave., Room 15307, San Francisco, California 94102 (415) 556-7487

San Francisco   211 Main St., 4th Floor, San Francisco, California 94105 (415) 556-0642

Fresno   2202 Monterey St., Room 108, Fresno, California 93721 (209) 487-5189

Sacramento   660 J Street, Room 215, Sacramento, California 95814 (916) 440-4461

Las Vegas   301 E. Stewart St., Las Vegas, Nevada 89125 (702) 388-6611

Reno   50 S. Virginia St., Room 238, Reno, Nevada 89505 (702) 784-5268

Honolulu   300 Ala Moana, Room 238, Honolulu, Hawaii 96850 (808) 546-8950

Agana   Pacific Daily News Bldg., Room 508, Agana, Guam 96910 (671) 472-7277
Los Angeles   350 S. Figueroa St., 6th Floor, Los Angeles, California 90071 (213) 894-2956
Santa Ana   2700 N. Main St., Room 400, Santa Ana, California 92701 (714) 836-2494
Phoenix   3030 N. Central Ave., Suite 1201, Phoenix, Arizona 85012 (602) 261-3732
Tucson   301 W. Congress St., Room 3V, Tucson, Arizona 85701 (602) 629-6715
San Diego   880 Front St., Room 4-S-29, San Diego, California (619) 293-5440

Region X

Seattle   2615 4th Ave., Room 440, Seattle, Washington 98121 (206) 442-5676
Seattle   915 Second Ave., Room 1792, Seattle, Washington 98174 (206) 442-5534
Anchorage   701 C St., Room 1068, Anchorage, Alaska 99501 (907) 271-4022
Fairbanks   101 12th Ave., Fairbanks, Alaska 99701 (907) 456-0211
Boise   1005 Main St., 2nd Floor, Boise, Idaho 83701 (208) 334-1696
Portland   1220 S. W. Third Ave., Room 676, Portland, Oregon 97204 (503) 221-2682
Spokane   W920 Riverside Ave., Room 651, Spokane, Washington 99210 (509) 456-3786

Department of Commerce

14th St. between Constitution and E Sts., NW,
Washington, DC 20230
(202) 377-2000

Background

The Department of Commerce encourages, serves, and promotes the nation's international and domestic interest in commerce. Because of the extremely wide scope of Commerce's responsibilities, a number of seemingly unrelated bureaus, administrations, and programs have been gathered under one roof. With the exception of the SBA, the range of programs and information available to the business community is unmatched elsewhere in the federal government.

Office of Business Liaison (OBL)
(202) 377-3176

The OBL offers business assistance through program information. Programs offered by all federal departments and agencies are covered in the OBL. The publication *Commerce Business Daily* includes most of the business opportunities available within the federal government (to order, refer to general information sources under Government Procurement below). When looking for assistance in dealing with the federal government, the OBL is a good place to start, as they inform department and administration officials of business community interests and critical issues.

The following program is offered in this area: Outreach Program, (202) 377-1360.

Census Bureau (202) 763-4100

The Census Bureau produces detailed statistical profiles of the nation which include information on population, housing, agriculture, manufacturing, transportation, construction, and the revenues and expenditures of state and local governments.

The following programs or services are offered in this area:

- Data user information
- Special tabulations and services

- Data user training
- Dissemination of statistical data

- Statistical abstracts

Bureau of Economic Analysis (BEA) (202) 523-0777

The BEA reports on the state of the U.S. economy and provides the technical information with which the gross national product is calculated. They also provide information on exports and imports. The data which is gathered by the BEA is available to the public in subscription magazines.

Office of Productivity, Technology and Innovation (OPTI) (202) 377-1984

The OPTI seeks to improve public policies for advancing private sector productivity, technological innovation, and business competitiveness. The OPTI identifies and eliminates barriers to productivity growth, provides assistance and information to businesses, works to strengthen incentives for the commercialization of federally funded research, and increases awareness of productivity-enhancing technologies and methods.

National Technical Information Service (NTIS) (703) 487-4600

The NTIS is a self-supporting information service organization within the Office of Productivity, Technology, and Innovation. It channels information concerning technological innovations and other specialized information to business, educators, government, and the public. Its products are intended to increase the efficiency and effectiveness of U.S. research and development and to support U.S. foreign policy goals by assisting the social and economic development of other nations. In return, U.S. access is increased to foreign technical information. For unusual or specific information needs, NTIS can produce a customized bibliography with abstracts of available material and information.

Economic Development Administration (EDA) (202) 377-5113

The EDA's purpose is to generate new jobs, to help protect existing jobs, to stimulate commercial and industrial growth in economically distressed areas of the United States, and to grant loan guarantees to industrial and commercial firms, local development companies, and Indian-owned enterprises. The loans may be used for working capital to maintain and expand operations for fixed assets such as land purchases, plant construction, and machinery or equipment purchases. Technical assistance and grants are available to enable communities and firms to find solutions to problems that stifle economic growth. Funds from the technical assistance program help businesses overcome a wide range of management and technical problems through university centers.

The following programs or services are offered in this area:

- Business development assistance
- Financial assistance
- Technical assistance

International Trade Administration (ITA) (202) 377-3808

The ITA assists American exporters in locating and gaining access to foreign markets and by furnishing information on foreign markets open to U.S. products and services.

The following programs or services are offered in this area:

- Export Counseling Office (202) 377-3181
- International markets services
- Agent distributor services
- Export contact list
- Major products

- Foreign buyers
- Business-sponsored promotions
- International trade fairs
- Video/catalog exhibitions
- Countervailing duty on imports
- Small trade missions
- International marketing information publications series
- New product information service
- Trade adjustment assistance

- Catalog exhibitions
- Overseas exhibitions
- Anti-dumping duties
- Interagency conferences on business export and investment
- District export councils
- Invest in the U.S.A.
- Product marketing service
- Seminars
- Trade complaints assistance
- Worldwide information and trade system

National Bureau of Standards (NBS) (202) 921-2318

The Bureau's overall goal is to strengthen and advance the nation's scientific and technological infrastructure and to facilitate its use for public benefit. The NBS is the only federal laboratory with the explicit goal of serving U.S. industry and science through the development of a wide variety of measurement services and participation in the development of standards.

The following programs or services are offered in this area:

- Research and technology applications
- Building science and technology
- Weights and measures services
- Calibration and testing services

Office of Consumer Affairs (202) 377-5001

The Office of Consumer Affairs provides advice and technical assistance to business on problems and issues of concern to consumers. Through services such as Customer Relations, businesses can better deal with consumer concerns such as advertising, warranties, handling of complaints, credit, and product safety.

Office of Small and Disadvantaged Business Utilization (OSDBU) (202) 377-3387

The OSDBU's primary responsibility is to help small and disadvantaged businesses achieve procurement goals. They also work closely with women, minorities, and firms in depressed areas.

Minority Business Development Agency (MBDA) (202) 377-1936

The MBDA was created to assist minority businesses in achieving effective and equitable participation in their attempts to overcome the social and economic disadvantages that have limited their past participation. Management and technical assistance are provided to these businesses upon request, primarily through a network of local business development organizations funded by MBDA.

The following programs or services are offered in this area:

- Bank development
- Business development organizations
- Business enterprise development
- Minority Business Opportunity Committee (MBOC)
- Construction contractor assistance
- Contract support services
- Capitol Hill assistance
- Research
- State and local government
- Federal procurement data service centers network

State Government

Overview

This section lists the primary agency or office in each state which provides excellent, one-stop guidance to the programs and services offered to small business on the state level. Under each listing, the specific areas of assistance available in each state are included. These agencies or offices are structured to meet the needs of individual firms either by providing direct assistance or by serving as an information clearing house. Each also has a working knowledge of federal and local opportunities for small business.

Function

Assistance and opportunities for small business are available in the following areas on a state-by-state basis.

Business Development

Start-up information on regulatory laws and permits; location selection assistance; demographic information; management training; bookkeeping; employee benefits and payroll administration; money management; technical and manufacturing assistance; labor and personnel training; high technology development.

Advocacy/Ombudsman Program. Person or office capable of walking a particular business through start-up, legislative and otherwise appropriate offices to get the business running; assists in solving regulatory and permitting problems faced by small businesses.

Managerial/Technical Assistance. Direct training and guidance on management and administrative practices; training and guidance on technical matters (e.g., manufacturing processes).

Training. Training services provided by the state, usually to promote employment in certain areas and industries.

Demographic Information. Statistics and analyses on population characteristics in specific geographic areas.

Enterprise Zones. Federally sponsored, state-administrated or locally sponsored/administrated programs in which tax incentives are given to promote business and to improve the local economy.

Financial Assistance

Guaranteed, direct, and revolving loans; grants; revenue bonds; information on venture capital sources; tax incentives.

Business Loan Program. A state sponsored or administered program to provide guaranteed, direct, or revolving loans to small businesses.

Venture Capital. Federally sponsored, state-administered effort to assist firms in obtaining seed money or up-front capital for promising small business projects.

Tax Incentives/Initiatives. Investment tax credits or reduction in state taxes to promote small business development.

Procurement Assistance

Assistance for marketing to state and local governments; set-aside contracts.

Small Business Program. Counseling for participation in state procurement, including assistance in the preparation of contracts. Set-Asides. A percentage of contracts reserved specifically for small and/or disadvantaged businesses.

These categories effectively cover the spectrum of small business needs, including start-up, expansion, locating sources of financing, personnel training, and more. This list, however, is not an exhaustive listing of all services that are offered on the state level. Contact with the state office regarding your specific needs and concerns may unveil additional services and assistance.

In some states, Small Business Development Centers (SBDCs) are listed in place of a solely state-sponsored agency. The SBDCs, co-sponsored by state universities and the U.S. Small Business Administration, serve as excellent information clearinghouses of available state programs for small business and also provide direct assistance in certain areas.

Almost all states publish information on services and assistance offered to small businesses in their state; however, the publications we have included in this section are outstanding as comprehensive resources to state services provided to small business. Again, a telephone call to the state office will reveal what is available in print.

Of course, all resources available to small businesses are available to minority and women-owned businesses. Some states, however, also give special consideration and offer special programs to these firms. The areas in which special programs are offered are listed under the heading "Minority/Women's Opportunities."

State Agencies

Alabama

Alabama Development Office, State Capitol,
Montgomery, AL 36130
(205) 263-0048

Business Development:
- Advocacy/ombudsman program
- Managerial/technical assistance
- Demographic information

Procurement Assistance:
- Small business program

Financial Assistance:
- Business loan program
- Venture capital

Minority/Women's Opportunities:
- Business loan program
- Venture capital
- Procurement assistance
- Set-asides
- Managerial/technical assistance
- Tax incentives/initiatives

Special Programs: High-technology development and expansion program.

Alaska

Office of Enterprise, Department of Commerce, Pouch D, Juneau, AK 99811
(907) 465-2018

Business Development:
- Advocacy/ombudsman program
- Managerial/technical assistance
- Demographic information

Procurement Assistance:
- Small business program
- Set-asides

Financial Assistance:
* Business loan program

Arizona

Office of Business and Trade, Department of Commerce,
1700 West Washington Street, 4th Floor, Phoenix, AZ 85007
(602) 255-5374

Business Development:
* Managerial/technical assistance
* Training
* Demographic information

Procurement Assistance:
* Small business program
* Set-asides

Arkansas

Small Business Development Center, University of Arkansas
(Little Rock), Library Building, Rm. 512, 33rd and University,
Little Rock, AR 72204
(501) 371-5381

Business Development:
* Advocacy/ombudsman program
* Managerial/technical assistance
* Demographic information
* Enterprise zone

Procurement Assistance:
* Small business program
* Set-asides

Financial Assistance:
* Business loan program

Minority/Women's Opportunities:
• Procurement assistance
• Set-asides
• Managerial/technical assistance

California

Office of Small Business Development, Department of Commerce, 1121 L St., Suite 600, Sacramento, CA 95814 (916) 445-6545

Business Development:
• Advocacy/ombudsman program
• Managerial/technical assistance
• Demographic information
• Enterprise zone

Procurement Assistance:
• Small business program
• Set-asides

Financial Assistance:
• Business loan program
• Venture capital program
• Tax incentives/initiatives

Special Programs: Revolving loan programs for high-tech industry expansion and development.

Colorado

Business Information Center, Office of Regulatory Reform, 1525 Sherman St., Rm. 110, Denver, CO 80203 (303) 866-3933

Business Development:
• Advocacy/ombudsman program
• Demographic information

Procurement Assistance:
• Small business program

Financial Assistance:
• Business loan program

Publications: *Doing Business in Colorado*

Connecticut

Small Business Services, Department of Economic
Development, 210 Washington St., Hartford, CT 06106
(203) 566-4051

Business Development:
• Advocacy/ombudsman program
• Managerial/technical assistance
• Demographic information
• Enterprise zone
• Training

Procurement Assistance:
• Small business program
• Set-asides
• Procurement assistance
• Set-asides

Financial Assistance:
• Business loan program
• Venture capital
• Tax incentives/initiatives

Minority/Women's Opportunities:
• Business loan program

Delaware

Economic Development Office, 99 King's Highway, P.O. Box 1401, Dover, DE 19903
(302) 736-4271

Business Development:
Advocacy/ombudsman program
• Demographic information
• Training
• Enterprise zone

Minority/Women Opportunities:
• Procurement assistance
• Set-asides
• Managerial/technical assistance
• Tax incentives/initiatives

Financial Assistance:
• Tax incentives/initiatives

Florida

Small Business Development Center, University of West Florida, Bldg. 8, Pensacola, FL 32514
(904) 474-2908

Business Development:
• Advocacy/ombudsman program
• Enterprise zone
• Managerial/technical assistance
• Demographic information

Procurement Assistance:
• Procurement assistance
• Set-asides

Financial Assistance:
• Venture capital

Minority/Women's Opportunities:
• Business loan program
• Venture capital
• Procurement assistance
• Set-asides
• Managerial/technical assistance

Special Programs: Department of Defense contracts available to small businesses listed with office.

Georgia

Small Business Development Center, 1180 East Broad St., Chicopee Complex, Athens, GA 30602
(404) 542-1721

Business Development:
• Advocacy/ombudsman program
• Managerial/technical assistance
• Demographic information
• Training

Procurement Assistance:
• Small business program
• Set-asides

Financial Assistance:
• Tax incentives/initiatives

Minority/Women's Opportunities:
• Business loan program
• Procurement assistance
• Set-asides

- Managerial/technical assistance
- Tax incentives/initiatives

Hawaii

Small Business Information Service, 250 South King St., Rm. 724, Honolulu, HI 96813
(808) 548-7645

Business Development:
- Advocacy/ombudsman program
- Managerial/technical assistance
- Demographic information
- Enterprise zone

Procurement Assistance:
- Small business program
- Set-asides

Financial Assistance:
- Business loan program
- Venture capital

Minority/Women's Opportunities:
- Business loan program
- Venture capital
- Procurement assistance
- Set-asides

Idaho

Division of Economic and Community Affairs, Department of Commerce, State Capitol, Rm. 108, Boise, ID 83720
(208) 334-2470

Business Development:
- Advocacy/ombudsman program

- Managerial/technical assistance
- Training
- Demographic information

Procurement Assistance:
- Small business program

Financial Assistance:
- Business loan program

Minority/Women's Opportunities:
- Procurement assistance

Special Programs: Regional small business revitalization loan programs.

Illinois

Bureau of Small Business, Department of Commerce and Community Affairs, 620 E. Adams St., Springfield, IL 62701 (217) 785-7500

Business Development:
- Advocacy/ombudsman program
- Managerial/technical assistance
- Demographic information
- Enterprise zone

Procurement Assistance:
- Small business program
- Set-asides
- Procurement assistance
- Managerial/technical assistance
- Tax incentives/initiatives

Financial Assistance:
- Business loan program

- Venture capital
- Tax incentives/initiatives

Minority/Women's Opportunities:
- Business loan program

Special Programs: One-stop center to start a small business

Indiana

Division of Business Expansion, Department of Commerce, Indiana Commerce Center, 1 N. Capital Ave., Suite 700, Indianapolis, IN 46204
(317) 232-8800

Business Development:
- Advocacy/ombudsman program
- Managerial/technical assistance
- Demographic information
- Enterprise zone

Procurement Assistance:
- Small business program
- Set-asides

Financial Assistance:
- Business loan program
- Venture capital
- Tax incentives/initiatives

Minority/Women's Opportunities:
- Procurement assistance
- Managerial/technical assistance

Special Programs: One-stop start-up service for new businesses.

Publications: *ORR/MUTZ: Economic Development Package*

Iowa

Small Business Division, Iowa Development Commission, 600 East Court Ave., Suite A, Des Moines, IA 50309
(505) 281-8310
(800) 532-1216 (In state)

Business Development
• Advocacy/ombudsman program
• Managerial/technical assistance

Procurement Assistance:
• Small business program

Financial Assistance:
• Business loan program
• Venture capital

Minority/Women's Opportunities:
• Procurement assistance
• Set-asides
• Managerial/technical assistance

Kansas

Small Business Development Center, Wichita State University, 021 Clinton Hall, Box 48, Wichita, KS 67208
(316) 689-3193

Business Development:
• Advocacy/ombudsman program
• Managerial/technical assistance
• Enterprise zone
• Demographic information

Procurement Assistance:
• Small business program

Financial Assistance:
• Business loan program
• Venture capital
• Tax incentives/initiatives

Minority/Women's Opportunities:
• Procurement assistance
• Set-asides

Kentucky

Business Information Clearinghouse, Commerce Cabinet
Capitol Plaza Tower, 22nd Floor, Frankfort, KY 40601
(502) 564-4252
(800) 626-2250

Business Development:
• Advocacy/ombudsman program
• Managerial/technical assistance
• Training
• Demographic information
• Enterprise zone

Procurement Assistance:
• Small business program
• Set-asides

Financial Assistance:
• Business loan program
• Venture capital
• Tax incentives/initiatives

Minority/Women's Opportunities:
• Procurement assistance
• Managerial/technical assistance

Special Programs: One step start-up program.

Louisiana

Small Business Specialist, Office of Commerce and Industry, 1 Maritime Plaza, P.O. Box 94185, Baton Rouge, LA 70802-9185 (504) 342-9224

Business Development:
• Advocacy/ombudsman program
• Managerial/technical assistance
• Training
• Demographic information
• Enterprise zone

Procurement Assistance:
• Small business program
• Set-asides

Financial Assistance:
• Business loan program
• Venture capital
• Tax incentives/initiatives

Minority/Women's Opportunities:
• Business loan program
• Venture capital
• Managerial/technical assistance

Publications: *Doing Business in Greater Baton Rouge*

Maine

Small Business Development Center, University of Southern Maine, 246 Deering Ave., Portland, ME 04102 (207) 780-4420

Business Development:
• Advocacy/ombudsman program

- Managerial/technical assistance
- Training
- Demographic information

Procurement Assistance:
- Small business program
- Set-asides

Financial Assistance:
- Business loan program
- Tax incentives/initiatives

Maryland

Office of Business and Industrial Development, Department of Economic and Community Development, 45 Calvert St., Annapolis, MD 21404
(301) 269-2945

Business Development:
- Advocacy/ombudsman program
- Managerial/technical assistance
- Training
- Demographic information
- Enterprise zone

Procurement Assistance:
- Small business program
- Set-asides

Financial Assistance:
- Business loan program

Minority/Women's Opportunities:
- Business loan program
- Procurement assistance
- Set-asides
- Tax incentives/initiatives

Special Programs: Economic Development Hotline: 1-800-OK-GREEN

Massachusetts

Small Business Assistance Division, Department of Commerce, 100 Cambridge St., 13th Floor, Boston, MA 02202
(617) 727-4005
(800) 632-8181 (In state)

Business Development:
• Managerial/technical assistance
• Training
• Demographic information
• Enterprise zone

Procurement Assistance:
• Small business program

Financial Assistance:
• Venture capital
• Tax incentives/initiatives
• Business loan program

Minority/Women's Opportunities:
• Procurement assistance
• Set-asides
• Managerial/technical assistance

Michigan

Local Development Service, Department of Commerce, P.O. Box 30225, Lansing, MI 48909
(517) 373-3530

Business Development:
• Advocacy/ombudsman program

- Managerial/technical assistance
- Training
- Demographic information

Procurement Assistance:
- Small business program

Financial Assistance:
- Business loan program
- Tax incentives/initiatives

Minority/Women's Opportunities:
- Business loan program
- Venture capital
- Procurement assistance
- Set-asides
- Managerial/technical assistance

Special Programs: Economic Development Hotline: 1-800-232-2727

Minnesota

Small Business Assistance Office, Department of Energy and Economic Development, 900 American Center, 150 E. Kellogg Blvd., St. Paul, MN 55107
(612) 296-3871

Business Development:
- Advocacy/ombudsman program
- Managerial/technical assistance
- Training
- Demographic information
- Enterprise zone

Procurement Assistance:
- Small business program
- Set-asides

Financial Assistance:
- Business loan program
- Venture capital
- Tax incentives/initiatives

Minority/Women's Opportunities:
- Procurement assistance
- Set-asides

Publications: *A Guide to Starting a Business in Minnesota*

Mississippi

Small Business Clearinghouse, Research and
Development Center, 3825 Ridgewood Rd.,
Jackson, MS 39211-6453
(601) 982-6231
(800) 521-7258 (In state)

Business Development:
- Advocacy/ombudsman program
- Managerial/technical assistance
- Training
- Demographic information
- Enterprise zone

Procurement Assistance:
- Small business program

Financial Assistance:
- Business loan program

Minority/Women's Opportunities:
- Set-asides

Publications: *Small Business Bibliography*

Missouri

Small Business Development Office, Division of
Community and Economic Development,
P.O. Box 118, Jefferson, City, MO 65102
(314) 751-4982

Business Development:
- Managerial/technical assistance
- Training
- Demographic information
- Enterprise zone

Financial Assistance:
- Business loan program
- Venture capital
- Tax incentives/initiatives

Minority/Women's Opportunities:
- Procurement assistance
- Managerial/technical assistance
- Tax incentives/initiatives

Publications: *Existing Business Resource Directory*

Montana

Business Assistance Division, Department of Commerce,
1424 Ninth Ave., Helena, MT 59620
(406) 444-3923

Business Development:
- Advocacy/ombudsman program
- Managerial/technical assistance
- Training
- Demographic information

Procurement Assistance:
- Set-asides

Financial Assistance:
• Business loan program
• Venture capital
• Tax incentives/initiatives

Minority/Women's Opportunities:
• Business loan program
• Venture capital
• Procurement assistance
• Set-asides
• Managerial/technical assistance
• Tax incentives/initiatives

Publications: *A Guide to Montana's Economic Development and Business Assistance Programs*

Nebraska

Small Business Division, Department of Economic Development, P.O. Box 94666, 301 Centennial Mall South, Lincoln, NE 68509
(402) 471-3111

Business Development:
• Advocacy/ombudsman program
• Managerial/technical assistance
• Training
• Demographic information

Procurement Assistance:
• Small business program

Financial Assistance:
• Business loan program
• Tax incentives/initiatives

Publications: *Resource for Nebraska Business*

Nevada

Small Business Development Center, University of Nevada, College of Business Administration, Business Building, Rm. 411, Reno, NV 89557-0016
(702) 784-1717

Business Development:
• Managerial/technical assistance
• Training
• Demographic information

Procurement Assistance
• Set-asides

Financial Assistance:
• Business loan program

Minority/Women's Opportunities:
• Procurement assistance

New Hampshire

Industrial Development Authority,
4 Park St., Room 302, Concord, NH 03301
(603) 721-2391

Business Development:
• Managerial/technical assistance
• Training
• Demographic information

Procurement Assistance:
• Small business program

Financial Assistance:
• Business loan program

Minority/Women's Opportunities:
- Venture capital

Publications: *Industrial New Hampshire*

New Jersey

Office of Small Business Assistance, Department of
Commerce and Economic Development,
1 West State St., CN 823, Trenton, NJ 08625
(609) 984-4442

Business Development:
- Advocacy/ombudsman program
- Managerial/technical assistance
- Training
- Demographic information
- Enterprise zone

Procurement Assistance:
- Small business program
- Set-asides

Financial Assistance:
- Business loan program
- Tax incentives/initiatives

Minority/Women's Opportunities:
- Business loan program
- Procurement assistance
- Set-asides
- Managerial/technical assistance

New Mexico

Business Development and Expansion, Department of
Economic Development and Tourism, Bataan Memorial Bldg.,

Suite 201, Santa Fe, NM 87503
(505) 827-6204

Business Development:
- Advocacy/ombudsman program
- Managerial/technical assistance
- Training
- Demographic information

Procurement Assistance:
- Small business program
- Set-asides

Financial Assistance:
- Business loan program
- Venture capital
- Tax incentives/initiatives

Minority/Women's Opportunities:
- Managerial/technical assistance

New York

Small Business Division, New York Department of Commerce, 230 Park Ave., Rm. 834, New York, NY 10169
(212) 309-0400

Business Development:
- Advocacy/ombudsman program
- Managerial/technical assistance
- Training
- Tax incentives/initiatives
- Demographic information

Procurement Assistance:
- Small business program
- Set-asides

Financial Assistance:
• Business loan program
• Venture capital

Minority/Women's Opportunities:
• Business loan program
• Venture capital
• Procurement assistance
• Set-asides
• Managerial/technical assistance
• Tax incentives/initiatives

Special Program: Small Business Advisory Board/Interagency Task Force Publications: *Your Business: A Management Guide for Small Business*

North Carolina

Small Business Development Division, Department of Commerce, Dobbs Bldg., Rm. 282, 430 N. Salisbury St., Raleigh, NC 27611 (919) 733-6254

Business Development:
• Advocacy/ombudsman program
• Managerial/technical assistance
• Training
• Demographic information
• Enterprise zone

Procurement Assistance:
• Small business program

Financial Assistance:
• Business loan program

Minority/Women's Opportunities:
• Procurement assistance

Publications: *A Directory of Services and Industry Offered by the State of North Carolina*

North Dakota

Small Business Specialist, Economic Development Commission, Liberty Memorial Bldg., Bismarck, ND 58505
(701) 224-2810

Business Development:
• Advocacy/ombudsman program
• Managerial/technical assistance
• Training
• Demographic information

Procurement Assistance:
• Small business program
• Set-asides

Financial Assistance:
• Business loan program
• Venture capital
• Tax incentives/initiatives

Special Programs: Center for Technology Transfer: mainframe computer access available to small engineering and architectural businesses.

Ohio

Small Business Office, Ohio Department of Development, P.O. Box 1001, Columbus, OH 43266-0101
(614) 466-4945
(800) 282-1085 (In state)

Business Development:
• Advocacy/ombudsman program

- Managerial/technical assistance
- Training
- Demographic information
- Enterprise zone

Procurement Assistance:
- Small business program
- Set-asides

Financial Assistance:
- Business loan program
- Tax incentives/initiatives

Minority/Women's Opportunities:
- Business loan program
- Procurement assistance
- Set-asides
- Managerial/technical assistance
- Tax incentives/initiatives

Oklahoma

Small Business Development Center, Station A,
517 West University, Durant, OK 74701
(405) 924-0277

Business Development:
- Advocacy/ombudsman program
- Managerial/technical assistance
- Training
- Demographic information

Procurement Assistance:
- Small business program
- Set-asides
- Managerial/technical assistance

Minority/Women's Opportunities:
• Business loan program
• Procurement assistance

Oregon

Oregon Economic Development Department,
595 Cottage Street, N.E., Salem, OR 97310
(503) 373-1200

Business Development:
• Managerial/technical assistance
• Training
• Demographic information
• Enterprise zone

Financial Assistance:
• Business loan program
• Venture capital
• Tax incentives/initiatives

Minority/Women's Opportunities
• Business loan program

Pennsylvania

Small Business Action Center, Department of Commerce,
483 Forum Bldg., Harrisburg, PA 17120
(717) 783-5700

Business Development:
• Advocacy/ombudsman program
• Managerial/technical assistance
• Training
• Tax incentives/initiatives
• Demographic information
• Enterprise zone

Procurement Assistance:
• Small business program
• Set-asides

Financial Assistance:
• Business loan program
• Venture capital

Minority/Women's Opportunities:
• Procurement assistance
• Managerial/technical assistance
• Set-asides

Publications: *Resource Directory for Small Business*

Rhode Island

Small Business Development Division,
Department of Economic Development,
7 Jackson Walkway, Providence, RI 02903
(401) 277-2601

Business Development:
• Advocacy/ombudsman program
• Managerial/technical assistance
• Training
• Demographic information

Procurement Assistance:
• Small business program
• Set-asides

Financial Assistance:
• Business loan program
• Tax incentives/initiatives

Minority/Women's Opportunities:
• Procurement assistance

Special Programs: Rhode Island Partnership of Service and Technology

South Carolina

Business Assistance Services and Information Center, Industry-Business and Community Services Division, State Development Board, P.O. Box 927, Columbia, SC 29202 (803) 758-3046

Business Development:
• Advocacy/ombudsman program
• Managerial/technical assistance
• Training
• Demographic information

Procurement Assistance:
• Small business program

Financial Assistance:
• Business loan program
• Tax incentives/initiatives

Minority/Women's Opportunities:
• Procurement assistance
• Set-asides
• Managerial/technical assistance
• Tax incentives/initiatives

Publications: *South Carolina Business Formation and Expansion Manual*

South Dakota

Small Business Development Center, University of South Dakota, 414 East Clark St., Vermillion, SD 57069-2390 (605) 677-5272

Business Development:
- Advocacy/ombudsman program
- Managerial/technical assistance
- Training
- Demographic information

Procurement Assistance:
- Small business program

Tennessee

Small Business Office, Department of Economic and Community Development, 320 6th Ave. North, 7th Floor, Rachel Jackson Bldg., Nashville, TN 37219
(615) 741-2626

Business Development:
- Advocacy/ombudsman program
- Managerial/technical assistance
- Training
- Demographic information

Procurement Assistance:
- Small business program
- Set-asides

Minority/Women's Opportunities:
- Procurement assistance
- Managerial/technical assistance

Publications: *A Guide to Doing Business in Tennessee*

Texas

Small and Minority Business Assistance Division, Economic Development Commission, P.O. Box 12728, Capitol Station, 410 East Fifth St., Austin, TX 78711
(512) 472-5059

Business Development:
- Advocacy/ombudsman program
- Managerial/technical assistance
- Training
- Demographic information

Procurement Assistance:
- Small business program
- Set-asides

Financial Assistance:
- Business loan program

Minority/Women's Opportunities:
- Business loan program
- Procurement assistance
- Managerial/technical assistance

Utah

Small Business Development Center, University of Utah, Business Classroom Bldg., Rm. 410-BUC, Salt Lake City, UT 84112 (801) 581-7905

Business Development:
- Advocacy/ombudsman program
- Managerial/technical assistance
- Training
- Demographic information

Procurement Assistance:
- Small business program
- Procurement assistance
- Managerial/technical assistance

Financial Assistance:
- Business loan program
- Venture capital

Minority/Women's Opportunities:
• Venture capital

Publications: *Doing Business in Utah*

Vermont

Small Business Development Center,
University of Vermont Extension Service,
Morrill Hall, Burlington, VT 05405
(802) 656-2990

Business Development:
• Managerial/technical assistance
• Training
• Demographic information

Procurement Assistance:
• Small business program

Financial Assistance:
• Business loan program

Minority/Women's Opportunities:
• Managerial/technical assistance
• Tax incentives/initiatives

Virginia

Small Business Coordinator, Department of Economic Development, 1000 Washington Building, Richmond, VA 23219
(804) 786-3791

Business Development:
• Advocacy/ombudsman program
• Managerial/technical assistance
• Training

- Demographic information
- Enterprise zone

Financial Assistance:
- Business loan program

Minority/Women's Opportunities:
- Procurement assistance

Publications: *Virginia Guide to Business Resources*

Washington

Small Business Development Center, 441 Todd Hall, Washington State University, Pullman, WA 99164 (509) 335-1576

Business Development:
- Advocacy/ombudsman program
- Managerial/technical assistance
- Training
- Demographic information
- Enterprise zone

Procurement Assistance:
- Small business program
- Set-asides

Financial Assistance:
- Business loan program
- Venture capital
- Tax incentives/initiatives

Minority/Women's Opportunities:
- Managerial/technical assistance

Special Program: Innovation Assessment Center

West Virginia

Small Business Division, Governor's Office of Community and Industrial Development, Capitol Complex, Charleston, WV 25305
(304) 348-2960

Business Development:
- Advocacy/ombudsman program
- Managerial/technical assistance
- Training
- Demographic information

Procurement Assistance:
- Set-asides

Financial Assistance:
- Business loan program
- Tax incentives/initiatives

Minority/Women's Opportunities:
- Business loan program
- Procurement assistance
- Managerial/technical assistance
- Tax incentives/initiatives

Wisconsin

Small Business Ombudsman, Department of Development, 123 W. Washington Ave., P.O. Box 7970, Madison, WI 53707
(608) 266-0562

Business Development:
- Advocacy/ombudsman program
- Managerial/technical assistance
- Training
- Demographic information
- Enterprise zone

Procurement Assistance:
- Small business program
- Set-asides

Financial Assistance:
- Business loan program
- Tax incentives/initiatives

Minority/Women's Opportunities:
- Set-asides
- Managerial/technical assistance
- Tax incentives/initiatives

Special Programs: 1-800-HELP BUSiness

Wyoming

Economic Development Division, Economic Development and Stabilization Board, Herschler Bldg., 3rd Floor East, Cheyenne, WY 82002
(307) 777-7287

Business Development:
- Managerial/technical assistance
- Demographic information

Procurement Assistance:
- Set-asides

Financial Assistance:
- Business loan program

Special Program: State Small Business Assistance Act

District of Columbia

Office of Business and Economic Development, District Bldg., Rm. 208, 1350 Pennsylvania Ave., N.W., Washington, DC 20004
(202) 727-6600

Business Development:
• Advocacy/ombudsman program
• Managerial/technical assistance
• Demographic information

Financial Assistance:
• Business loan program
• Venture capital

Minority/Women's Opportunities:
• Procurement assistance
• Set-asides

APPENDIX C

State Locator Telephone Numbers of Key Federal Offices[a]

State	IRS[b]	Commerce	OSHA	FICs	
Alabama	(205) 254-0403 Birmingham	(205) 254-1331	(205) 822-7100 Birmingham	322-8591[c]	Birmingham
			(205) 690-2131 Mobile	438-1421[c]	Mobile
Alaska	(907) 561-7484	(907) 271-5041	(907) 271-5152	(907) 271-3650	Anchorage
Arizona	(602) 261-3861	(602) 261-3285	(602) 241-2006	(602) 261-3313	Phoenix
				(602) 261-3313	Tucson
Arkansas	(501) 378-5685	(501) 378-5794	(501) 378-6291	378-6177[c]	Little Rock
California	(415) 556-0880 San Francisco	(415) 556-5860 San Francisco	(213) 432-3434 Long Beach	(213) 894-3800	Los Angeles

(continues)

State	IRS[b]	Commerce	OSHA	FICs
	(213) 894-4574 Los Angeles		(415) 556-7260 San Francisco	(916) 551-2380 Sacramento (619) 293-6030 San Diego (415) 556-6600 San Francisco 836-2632[c] Santa Ana
Colorado	(303) 825-7041	(303) 844-3246	(303) 844-5258	(303) 236-7181 Denver 471-9491[c] Colorado Springs 544-9523[c] Pueblo
Connecticut	(203) 722-3064 Hartford	(203) 722-3530	(203) 722-2294	527-2617[c] Hartford 624-4720[c] New Haven
Delaware	(302) 573-6400	(215) 597-2866 Phila., PA		
Florida	(904) 791-2514 Jacksonville	(305) 536-5267 Miami (904) 488-6469 Tallahassee (904) 791-2796 Jacksonville	(305) 527-7292 Ft. Lauderdale (813) 228-2821 Tampa (904) 791-2895 Jacksonville	522-8531[c] Ft. Lauderdale 354-4756[c] Jacksonville (305) 536-4155 Miami 422-1800[c] Orlando (813) 893-3495 St. Petersburg 229-7911[c] Tampa 833-7566[c] West Palm Beach
Georgia	(404) 221-3808	(912) 944-4205 Savannah (404) 881-7000 Atlanta	(404) 939-8987 Tucker (912) 233-3923 Savannah	(404) 221-6891 Atlanta
Hawaii	(808) 546-8660	(808) 546-8694	(800) 546-3157	(808) 546-8620 Honolulu
Idaho	(208) 334-1328 Boise	(503) 221-3001 Portland, OR		
Illinois	(312) 886-4669 Chicago (217) 492-4288 Springfield	(312) 353-4450	(312) 891-3800 Calumet City (312) 896-8700 North Aurora (309) 671-7033 Peoria (312) 631-8200 Niles	(312) 353-4242
Indiana	(317) 269-6326 Indianapolis	(317) 269-6214	(317)269-7290	883-4110[c] Gary/Hammond (317) 269-7373 Indianapolis

Iowa	(515) 284-4870 Des Moines	(515) 284-4222 Des Moines	(515) 281-3606 Des Moines	(800) 532-1556
Kansas	(316) 263-6112 Wichita	(816) 374-3142 K.C., MO	(316) 269-6644	
Kentucky	(502) 582-6259 Louisville	(502) 582-5066	(502) 564-6895	(502) 582-6261 Louisville
Louisiana	(504) 589-2801 New Orleans	(504) 589-6546	(504) 342-3126 Baton Rouge	(504) 589-6696 New Orleans
Maine	(800) 225-0717		(203) 722-2294 Hartford, CT (207) 622-8417	
Maryland	(301) 962-2222 Baltimore	(301) 962-3560	(301) 962-2840	(301) 962-4980
Massachusetts	(617) 223-5177 Boston	(617) 223-2312	(617) 647-8681 Waltham (413) 785-0123 Springfield	(617) 223-7121
Michigan	(313) 226-3671	(313) 226-3650	(313) 226-6720	(313) 226-7016 Detroit 451-2628ᶜ Grand Rapids
Minnesota	(806) 652-9062 (612) 725-7320 St. Paul	(612) 349-3338 Minneapolis	(612) 296-2116	(612) 349-5333 Minneapolis
Mississippi	(601) 960-4526 Jackson	(601) 960-4388	(601) 982-6315	
Missouri	(314) 425-5660	(314) 425-3302 St. Louis (816) 374-3142 Kansas City	(816) 374-2756 Kansas City (314) 263-2749 St. Louis	(314) 425-4106 (314) 425-4106 St. Louis
Montana	(406) 449-5392 Helena		(406) 657-6649	
Nebraska	(402) 221-3501 Omaha	(402) 221-3664 Omaha	(402) 221-3182 Omaha	(402) 221-3353 Omaha
Nevada	(702) 784-5521 Reno (702) 388-6291 Las Vegas	(702) 784-5203 Reno	(702) 789-0380 Reno	
New Hampshire	(603) 436-7720 Ext. 772	(617) 223-2312 Boston, MA	(603) 224-1995	
New Jersey	(201) 645-6478	(609) 989-2100	(201) 359-2777 Belle Mead (201) 288-1700 Hasbrouk Hts. (609) 657-6808 Camden (201) 361-4050 Dover	(201) 645-3600 Newark 396-4400ᶜ Trenton
New Mexico		(505) 766-2386	(505) 766-3411	(505) 766-3091 Albuquerque
New York	(212) 264-3310 N.Y.C. (718) 596-3610	(716) 846-4191 Buffalo (212) 264-0634 N.Y.C.	(212) 264-9840 N.Y.C. (518) 472-6085 Albany (315) 423-5188 Syracuse (716) 454-3710 Rochester	463-4421ᶜ Albany (716) 846-4010 Buffalo (212) 264-4464 N.Y.C. 546-5075ᶜ Rochester

(continues)

State	IRS[b]	Commerce	OSHA	FICs
			(914) 997-9510 White Plains (716) 684-5145 Buffalo (516) 334-3344 Westbury	476-8545[c] Syracuse
North Carolina	(919) 378-5620 Greensboro		(919) 856-4770 Raleigh	376-3600[c] Charlotte
North Dakota	(701) 237-5771 Ext. 5105 Fargo	(402) 221-3664 Omaha, NE	(701) 255-4011 Ext. 521	
Ohio	(216) 522-3414 Cleveland (513) 684-2828 Cincinnati	(513) 684-2944 Cincinnati (216) 522-4750 Cleveland	(216) 522-3818 Cleveland (513) 684-3784 Cincinnati (614) 469-5582 Columbus (419) 259-7542 Toledo	375-5638[c] Akron (513) 684-2801 Cincinnati (216) 522-4040 Cleveland 221-1014[c] Columbus 241-3223[c] Toledo
Oklahoma	(918) 583-5121 Tulsa	(405) 231-5302 Okla. City	(405) 231-5351 Okla. City	(405) 231-4868 Okla. City 584-4193[c] Tulsa
Oregon	(503) 221-3960 Portland	(503) 221-3001 Portland	(503) 221-2251 Portland	(503) 221-2222 Portland
Pennsylvania	(412) 644-6504 Pittsburgh (215) 597-0512 Philadelphia	(215) 597-2866 Philadelphia (412) 644-2850 Pittsburgh	(412) 644-2905 Pittsburgh (215) 597-4955 Philadelphia (717) 826-6538 Wilkes Barre (717) 782-3902 Harrisburg (814) 453-4351 Erie	(215) 597-7042 Philadelphia (412) 644-3456 Pittsburgh 346-7081[c] Scranton
Rhode Island	(401) 528-4276 Providence	(401) 277-2605	(401) 528-4669 Providence	331-5565[c] Providence
South Carolina	(803) 253-3032 Columbia	(803) 765-5345 Columbia	(803) 765-5904 Columbia	
South Dakota	(605) 225-0250 Aberdeen Ext. 262	(402) 221-3664 Omaha, NE		
Tennessee	(615) 259-4601 Nashville	(615) 251-5161 Nashville (901) 521-4826 Memphis	(615) 251-5313 Nashville	242-5056[c] Nashville (901) 521-3285 Memphis 265-8231[c] Chattanooga
Texas	(512) 472-1974 Austin	(214) 767-0542 Dallas	(713) 222-4305 Houston	472-5494[c] Austin

State	IRS	Commerce	OSHA	FICs
	(713) 954-6878 Houston (214) 767-1428 Dallas	(512) 482-5783 Austin (214) 767-5347 Irving		(817) 334-3624 Ft. Ward (713) 229-2552 Houston 224-4471[c] San Antonio 767-8585[c] Dallas
Utah		(801) 524-5116 Salt Lake City	(801) 524-5080 Salt Lake City	(801) 524-5353 Salt Lake City
Vermont	(802) 951-6370 Burlington	(617) 223-2312 Boston	(603) 224-1995	
Virginia	(804) 771-2289 Richmond	(804) 771-2246 Richmond	(804) 786-5873 Richmond	(804) 441-3101 Norfolk 643-4928[c] Richmond 982-8591[c] Roanoke
Washington	(206) 442-5515 Seattle	(206) 442-5615 Seattle	(206) 442-7520 Seattle	(206) 442-0570 Seattle 383-5230[c] Tacoma
West Virginia	(304) 420-6600	(304) 347-5123	(304) 347-5937	
Wisconsin	(414) 291-3302 Milwaukee	(414) 291-3473 Milwaukee	(414) 291-3315 Milwaukee	
Wyoming	(307) 772-2162 Cheyenne	(303) 837-3246 Denver, CO	(303) 844-5285	
Washington, DC	(202) 488-3100	(202) 377-2000	(202) 523-9361	(202) 655-4000

[a]Abbreviations: IRS, Internal Revenue Service; Commerce, U.S. Department of Commerce; OSHA, Occupational Safety and Health Administration; FICs, Federal Information Centers.

[b]The IRS toll-free number for all states, except those otherwise listed, is (800) 424-1040.

[c]Indicates telephone number for use only within the city indicated.

Small Business Development Centers

The 46 Small Business Development Centers listed in this section cover 41 states, the District of Columbia, Puerto Rico, and the Virgin Islands. For an explanation of the function of SBDCs, see Appendix A. Contact the SBDC nearest you for assistance.

Region I

University of Southern Maine   246 Deering Avenue, Portland, Maine 04102 (207) 780-4423

University of Massachusetts   School of Management, Amherst, Maine 01003 (413) 549-4930

University of Connecticut   368 Fairfield Rd., SBA U-41, Room 422, Storrs, Connecticut 06268 (203) 486-4135

Bryant College   Smithfield, Rhode Island 02917 (401) 232-6000

University of Vermont   Extension Service, Morrill Hall, Burlington, Vermont 05405 (802) 656-4479

University of New Hampshire   110 McConnell Hall, Durham, New Hampshire 03824 (603) 862-3558

Region II

Rutgers University   Ackerson Hall-3rd Floor, 180 University Ave., Newark, New Jersey 07102 (201) 648-5950

State University of New York   State University Plaza, Albany, New York 12246 (518) 473-5398
College of the Virgin Islands   P.O. Box 1087, St. Thomas, Virgin Islands 00802 (809) 776-3206
University of Puerto Rico   Mayaguez Campus, Mayaguez, Puerto Rico 00709 (809) 834-4040

Region III

University of Pennsylvania   University City Science Center, 2440 Market St., Suite 202 Philadelphia, Pennsylvania 19104-3306 (215) 898-1219
Howard University   2600 6th St., N.W. Room 128, Washington, DC 20059 (202) 636-5150
University of Charleston   2300 MacCorkle Ave., SE, Charleston, West Virginia 25304 (304) 357-4800
University of Delaware   Suite 005-Purnell Hall, Newark, Delaware 19711 (302) 451-2747

Region IV

University of South Carolina   College of Business Administration, Columbia, South Carolina 29208 (803) 777-4907
University of West Florida   State Coordinators Office, Bldg. 38, Room 107, Pensacola, Florida 32514 (904) 474-3016
University of Alabama in Birmingham   School of Business, 1717 11th Ave. South, Suite 419 Birmingham, Alabama 35294 (205) 934-7260
University of Georgia   1180 E. Broad St., Chicopee Complex, Athens, Georgia 30602 (404) 542-5760
University of Kentucky   18 Porter Bldg., Lexington, Kentucky 40506-0205 (606) 257-1751
University of Mississippi   3825 Ridgewood Rd., Jackson, Mississippi 39211 (601) 982-6760
Memphis State University   3876 Central Ave., Memphis, Tennessee 38152 (901) 454-2500

University of North Carolina   820 Clay St., Raleigh, North Carolina 27605 (919) 733-4643

Region V

University of Wisconsin   602 State St., Second Floor, Madison, Wisconsin 53703 (608) 263-7794

College of St. Thomas   1107 Hazeltine Blvd., Suite 452, Chaska, Minnesota 55318 (612) 448-8810

Wayne State University   2727 Second Ave., Detroit, Michigan 48201 (313) 577-4848

Department of Commerce and Community Affairs   620 East Adams St., Springfield, Illinois 62701 (217) 785-6174

Indiana Economic Development Council   One North Capitol, Suite 200, Indianapolis, Indiana 46204 (317)634-6407

Region VI

University of Arkansas   Library Bldg., 5th Floor, 33rd & University Ave., Little Rock, Arkansas 72204 (501) 371-5381

Northeast Louisiana University   Administration 2-99, College of Business, Monroe, Louisiana 71209 (318) 342-2464

University of Texas at Arlington   College of Engineering, P.O. Box 19209, Arlington, Texas 76019-0029 (817) 273-2559

Southeastern Oklahoma State University   Station A, Box 4194, Durant, Oklahoma 74701 (405) 924-0277

University of Houston   University Park, Suite 127 Heyne Bldg., 4800 Calhoun Rd., Houston, Texas 77004 (713) 749-4236

Region VII

University of Nebraska at Omaha   Peter Kiewit Center, Omaha, Nebraska 68182 (402) 554-2521

Iowa State University   205 Engineering Annex, Ames, Iowa 50011 (515) 294-3420

St. Louis University   3642 Lindell Blvd., St. Louis, Missouri 63108 (314) 534-7232
Wichita State University   021 Clinton Hall, Box 48, Wichita, Kansas 67208 (316) 689-3193

Region VIII

University of Utah   420 Chipeta Way, Suite 110, Salt Lake City, Utah 84108 (801) 581-4869
University of South Dakota   Business Research Bureau, 414 E. Clarke St., Vermillon, South Dakota 57069-2390 (605) 677-5272
Casper Community College   944 East Second St., Casper, Wyoming 82601 (307) 235-4825
University of North Dakota   College of Business & Public Administration, Box 8098, Grand Forks, North Dakota 58202 (701) 780-3120

Region IX

University of Nevada Reno   College of Business Administration, Rm. 411, Reno, Nevada 89557-0016 (702) 784-1717
Department of Commerce   State of California, 1121 L St., Suite 600, Sacramento, California 95814 (916) 324-8102

Region X

Washington State University   441 Todd Hall, Pullman, Washington 99164-4740 (509) 335-1576
Lane Community College   Downtown Center, 1059 Willamette St., Eugene, Oregon 97401 (503) 726-0250

Selected Business Organizations

Chamber of Commerce of the United States

1615 H St., NW, Washington, DC 20062
(202) 659-6000

The Chamber of Commerce is organized at the local, state, and national levels.

Local Chambers meet the needs and desires of the local business community with various programs in economic development, community and human resources, and public affairs. Specific programs often found at the local level include:

- Small business development
- Group courses and seminars on management led by professionals or practitioners
- Group and individual counseling on small business problems
- Start-up assistance, lending, and equity capital programs

State Chambers coordinate local Chamber programs statewide and represent the state business community to the state government. Information is available through the state Chamber on small business programs in the state.

The national Chamber, the Chamber of Commerce of the U.S., works with developing local and state chambers and represents national business interests to the federal government.

The Small Business Programs Office acts as a central clearinghouse for information on everything from getting started in business to expanding your business overseas. Available resources include:

- *U.S. Chamber Information Resources Guide.* Lists U.S. Chamber publications, guides, filmstrips, and slide shows for small business.
- *The State and Local Chamber Lists.* Complete lists of state and local Chambers that have small business and export assistance programs.

Chamber staff specialists provide information, opinions, and analysis in several areas of importance to small business. For a copy of their names and telephone numbers, along with specialty areas, contact (301) 468-5128 and ask for the *U.S. Chamber Staff Specialists* brochure. Areas of interest include:

- Legislation
- Regulations (e.g., environmental control, job safety, health, labor law, etc.)
- Statistical information (e.g., economic aggregates, industry breakdowns, forecasts, etc.)
- International trade (e.g., export/import rules and regulations, foreign market information, etc.)
- Federal government procurement
- Tax laws and regulations

The National Federation of Independent Business (NFIB)

150 West 20th Ave., San Mateo, CA 94403 (headquarters)
(415) 341-7441
600 Maryland Ave., SW, Suite 700, Washington, DC 20024
(202) 554-9000

Background

As the nation's largest organization representing small and independent businesses, the NFIB represents more than 500,000 business owners in the legislatures as well as with state and federal agencies. The NFIB also disseminates education information on free enterprise, entrepreneurship, and small business.

Services

- Provides surveys on economic trends
- Provides studies on a broad range of information pertinent to businesses
- Lobbies for small business members on particular issues
- Provides entrepreneurship educational materials
- Holds conferences and membership meetings

Publications

- *NFIB Mandate.* Explains legislative actions of NFIB lobbyists; sent monthly to members
- *How Congress Voted.* Printed for each Congressional term, describes the trends of voting in Congress and provides a rundown, by state, of the voting on NFIB issues by members of Congress
- *NFIB Legislative Priorities.* Published before each session of Congress to expound the position of the NFIB on issues related to small business

• *Action Report*. Comes out each session of Congress and reports on positions taken by the NFIB

National Small Business Association (NSBA)

1604 K St., NW, Washington, DC 20006
(202) 293-8830

Background

A membership-based association of business owners representing all types of business, the NSBA presents small businesses' point of view to all levels of government and the Congress. The NSBA also develops programs of national policy that are of concern to the small business community.

Services

• Provides members with a monthly newsletter and other materials which keep them up-to-date on issues affecting their businesses
• Members are alerted to federal contracting opportunities through the Bidder's Early Alert Message system

Small Business United (SBU)

69 Hickory Drive, Waltham, MA 02154
(617) 890-9070

Background

A network of regional small business organizations, the SBU was formed in 1981 to represent these organizations and the concerns of small business before lawmakers. It works regularly with Congressional and Executive Branch officials in Washington and the field.

SBU offers no direct services to small business in particular; rather it is a networking organization. Direct services are offered by member organizations which are listed below.

Member Organizations

Located in various parts of the country, SBU's member organizations work at the regional level to serve the needs of small business. They are diverse in orientation and in services provided. Services include:

- Management assistance
- Educational programs
- Troubleshooting for common business problems
- Counseling
- Regional networking information
- Promotion of regional small business interests

Many provide important publications that provide key regional information. Contact the organization nearest you. Following is a listing of these organizations.

The Smaller Business Association of New England (SBANE)
69 Hickory Drive, Waltham, Massachusetts 02154 (617) 890-9070
(800) 368-6803
(Operates in the New England area)

The Smaller Manufacturers Council (SMC)
339 Boulevard of the Allies, Pittsburgh, Pennsylvania 15222
(412) 391-1622
(Operates in the tristate area of western Pennsylvania, eastern Ohio, northern West Virginia)

Independent Business Association of Wisconsin (IBA)
415 East Washington Ave., East Madison, Wisconsin 53703 (608)
251-5546
(Operates in Wisconsin)

Council of Smaller Enterprise (COSE)
690 Huntington Building, Cleveland, Ohio 44115 (216) 621-3300
(Operates in Greater Cleveland and surrounding region)

Small Business Association of Michigan (SBAM)
490 West South Street, Kalamazoo, Michigan 49007 (616) 342-2400
(Operates in Michigan)

Texas Association of Small Business Councils (TASC)
Greater Chamber of Commerce, P.O. Box 1628,
San Antonio, Texas 78926 (512) 366-0099
(Operates in Texas)

Independent Business Association of Illinois (IBAIL)
8565 W. Dempster, Suite 200, Niles, Illinois 60648 (312) 692-7306
(Operates in Illinois)

Ohio Small Business Council (OSBC)
Ohio Chamber of Commerce, 35 E. Gay Street,
Columbus, Ohio 43215 (614) 228-4201
(Operates in Ohio)

National Association of Manufacturers (NAM)

1776 F St., NW, Washington, DC 20006
(202) 637-3046

Background

A membership-based association of 13,000 manufacturing firms, more than 9,000 of which have fewer than 500 employees. Member firms account for 80% of the nation's industrial capacity.

The voice for the manufacturing community in Washington, NAM provides members with an opportunity to participate in the public policy process through membership on 14 policy committees. Major subject areas include:

- Resource and technology (energy, environment, innovation, natural resources)
- International economic affairs (international investment, finance, and trade)
- Industrial relations (labor relations, human resources, employee benefits, loss prevention and control)
- Government regulation, competition, and small manufacturing
- Taxation and fiscal policy

Services

One hundred subject specialists (legislative specialists, lawyers, communications advisors, and public affairs experts) help members with questions and problems. The *NAM Member Service Guide* provides the names and telephone numbers of these specialists.

Publications

Enterprise. NAM's monthly magazine, probes current and emerging issues in articles written by industry experts and national figures.

American Entrepreneurs Association

2311 Pontius Ave., Los Angeles, CA 90064
(213) 478-0437

Background

The American Entrepreneurs Association is a membership-based organization which helps and inspires people to enter the world of entrepreneurship.

Services

- Offers more than 250 extensive start-up operations manuals which are available for purchase, each of which contains complete step-by-step instructions necessary to start and run a business.
- Offers members discounts on the operations manuals and free counseling; they also receive the monthly magazine *Entrepreneur*. [To become a member, call (800) 421-2300 or (800) 852-7449 in California.]

Publications

- *Entrepreneur*. A monthly magazine with feature articles of interest to small business owners.
- *Choices for Entrepreneurial Women*. A quarterly magazine oriented toward helping women entrepreneurs expand their businesses.

National Association of Development Companies (NADC)

1612 K St., NW, Suite 706, Washington, DC 20006
(202) 785-8484

Background

The National Association of Development Companies is a joint government/private sector program organized in 1981 to represent the Certified Development Companies participating in SBA lending programs for small businesses established by Section 503 of the Small Business Investment Act. Certified Development Companies are established by local development agencies to provide SBA, private, and bank funds for economic development.

The NADC provides long-term fixed-asset financing to eligible small businesses.

Services

- Offers training and technical assistance
- Acts as a liaison with Members of Congress and SBA officials
- Runs an annual membership conference

Publications

NADCO News. Published monthly and free to members; covers SBA developments, events of interest to small business operators, and federal events information.

National Association of Entrepreneurs

2378 S. Broadway, Denver, CO 80210
(303) 440-3322

Background

The National Association of Entrepreneurs helps to increase the longevity of new and developing small businesses by networking resources and small business operators to exchange ideas, information, and support. Local chapters of the NAE are chartered in population centers of 25,000 or more. If there is no local chapter in your area and you would like to start one, contact the NAE.

Services

- Monthly meetings provide interactive format for networking and the exchange of information

- Telephone help line for members (task force service)
- Various workshops and seminars designed to improve managerial skills, with accompanying booklets and tapes
- Annual national entrepreneur conference

Publications

NAE Journal. Contains articles of interest to small business operators as well as advice on managerial assistance.

National Association of Small Business Investment Companies (NASBIC)

1156 15th St., NW, Suite 1101, Washington, DC 20005
(202) 833-8230

Background

The NASBIC coordinates and promotes activities of over 400 small business investment companies (SBICs) nationwide. SBICs are privately capitalized, owned, and managed investment firms licensed by the SBA that provide equity capital, long-term financing, and management assistance to small businesses. SBICs can borrow funds from the government on a long-term basis for reinvestment in small businesses. The SBIC program emphasizes investment in the small growth firms that generate jobs.

Services

Assistance provided by individual SBICs (see publications below).

Publications

- *Venture Capital: Where to Find It.* Available from NASBIC for $1.00 and a self-addressed, stamped business enve-

lope (use above address). The 28-page directory lists over 400 SBICs and MESBICs (Minority Enterprise SBICs).
• *Capital-Raising References for Small Business*. Lists directories, books, booklets, periodicals and newsletters available.

National Association of Women Business Owners (NAWBO)

221 N. La Salle St., Suite 2026, Chicago, IL 60601
(312) 346-2330

Background

The National Association of Women Business Owners is a membership-based federation with 27 local chapters and 2400 members nationwide. NAWBO works with women business owners to expand their operations and represents women's business interests to federal and state governments.

Services

• Provides counseling and technical assistance at the local level, primarily through networking with local members.
• Holds monthly programs at the local chapters which address women business owner problems
• Annual national conference provides management and technical assistance training through workshops and seminars

American Association of Minority Enterprise Small Business Investment Companies (MESBICs)

915 15th St., NW, Suite 700, Washington, DC 20005
(202) 347-8600

Background

The American Association of Minority Enterprise Small Business Investment Companies is a trade association representing an industry of investment companies that invest exclusively in small businesses owned by socially or economically disadvantaged entrepreneurs.

Most MESBICs are also members of the National Association of Small Business Investment Companies (NASBIC) (see separate listing).

Services

• Provides entrepreneurs with the names of investors in their area
• A national directory of MESBICs is available for $3.39

National Business League (NBL)

4324 Georgia Ave., NW, Washington, DC 20011
(202) 829-5900

Background

Established in 1900 with the goal of achieving economic independence, the NBL is a national federation with membership in 37 states and 127 local chapters. Primarily involved in business development among blacks, it serves as a voice for black business on Capitol Hill and in the federal government. The NBL works to expand minority business participation in franchise ownership and operation, especially in fast-food and auto-related industries, but also in transportation, telecommunications, high-tech, and energy-related fields.

Services

• Provides assistance for black small businesses; problems are assessed and referrals made, especially in the areas of

capital formation and minority set-aside programs
• Offers educational opportunities through workshop training at NBL institutes and seminar programs

Publications

The National Memo, Briefs, and the *Corporate Guide for Minority Vendors.*

U.S. Hispanic Chamber of Commerce

829 Southwest Blvd., Kansas City, MO 64108
(816) 842-2228

Background

As the only national Hispanic business association, the Chamber represents the interests of over 400,000 Hispanic-owned firms. The Chamber advocates the business interests of Hispanics and develops minority business opportunities with major corporations and all levels of government. Its annual convention combines trade fair, business sections, and workshops designed to promote Hispanic business opportunities.

Services

• Network capabilities with over 200 Chambers nationwide
• Referral service linking small business persons with government or corporate procurement agents
• Training and technical assistance for procurement business opportunities

Publications

Quarterly newsletter and bulletin; annual magazine.